# LABORATORY MANUAL FOR CLINICAL VETERINARY TECHNOLOGY

Oreta Marie Samples, BS, RVT, MPH, DHSc

M. Scott Echols, DVM, Dipl ABVP

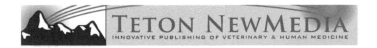

TETON NEWMEDIA
INNOVATIVE PUBLISHING OF VETERINARY & HUMAN MEDICINE

Executive Editor: Carroll C. Cann

Teton NewMedia
5286 Dunewood Dr,
Florence, OR 97439
541.991.3342
www.tetonnm.com

The author and publisher have made every effort to provide an accurate reference text. However, they shall not be held responsible for problems arising from errors or omissions, or from misunderstandings on the part of the reader.

ISBN # 978-1-59161-051-9
Print number 5 4 3 2 1

Library of Congress Cataloging-in-Publication Data on file.

**Supplementary Resources for Instructors Only Disclaimer:**
Additional resources were made available for this title for instructors of the text only. Instructors can find these resources available here: https://resourcecentre.routledge.com/books/9781591610519

# PREFACE

The study of clinical pathology is more pertinent than ever for veterinary technology students due to the vast number of disease-causing organisms that affect domestic animals and sometimes their human caretakers. This is especially true with companion animals who are not only "owned" by humans, they are cherished and regarded as family members sharing close bonds. This closeness can lead to shared infections and other diseases which are capable of animal to human transmission.

In developing this laboratory manual, the authors have attempted to provide a learning resource that aligns with the AVMA-CVTEA recommended skills and tasks which technician students must master. Additionally, we hope to challenge the student to think critically about the animals that they interact with, the symptomatology that is presented to them and how this relates to the diagnosis, treatment and care of the patient. We are not suggesting that technicians should engage in diagnosing or preparing treatment plans. Veterinary technical and nursing staff should, however, be able to understand and facilitate the collection of specimens for in-house and/or referred testing, and carry out an appropriate treatment plan in order to provide the clinician with information that will make his job easier and facilitate a positive outcome for the patient.

The relationship humans have with animals spans many fields and includes companion, food, zoo, aviary, aquaria, research, wildlife and more. Management and care for such diversity in species and situations often requires a team effort – of which the veterinary technical and nursing staff are a critical component. It is with great respect for veterinary support staff that we present this manual.

**Oreta M. Samples, BS, RVT, MPH, DHSc**
**M. Scott Echols, DVM, Dipl. ABVP**

# ACKNOWLEDGEMENT

This manual has been a labor of love that began 24 years ago when I first began working as an academic veterinary technician at a small veterinary technology program in Georgia at a time when there were no lab manuals to guide our studies. I would like to acknowledge Dr. Kashmiri Arora who challenged me to take charge of the clinical pathology laboratory in 1995 and find resources. Failing to find these resources, he allowed me free reign to create my own. What you have is a 24-year labor of love offered to all veterinary technician students both in the past and the future for their educational benefit. Thanks Dr. Arora….it was well worth it. I would also like to thank Dr. Custin Ben Lowery who was my mentor throughout the program, without him, I would not be the professional that I am today. Dr. Frederick McLaughlin deserves a great shout-out for his patience in teaching a myopic, astigmatism-plagued student that blood cells were not moving and that there were not 3 million of them on the slide; your patience in helping me adjust for my own disabilities knew no bounds and I am forever grateful. I think of you every time I peer into a microscope. A special thank you to Dr. S. Mobini and to Dr. George McCommon who at various times were my Department Head and allowed me the freedom to work on this project. Your faith in my abilities sometimes outshone my own, thank you for everything.

**Oreta M. Samples, BS, RVT, MPH, DHsc**

The veterinary profession is not complete and would suffer greatly without the active participation and contributions of veterinary technicians and support staff. I have relied upon and learned from numerous veterinary nurses throughout my career. Their observations and care have helped save lives, and in many cases, guided my diagnostic and therapeutic decisions. My mentor and friend Dr. Brian Speer initially taught me the true value of support staff during my formative days as a resident in avian medicine and surgery. Since then, I have learned to listen to the nursing staff and help support them in their career. Over the years and while working in several hospitals I have had the pleasure of interacting with numerous outstanding men and women who call themselves technicians or nurses. I would like to recognize Crystal Wilcox, LVT, Melisa King-Smith (now Dr. King-Smith) and Jill Murray, RVT, RLATG, VTS (Exotic Companion Animal) who directly contributed photos for this manual. To my family, my wife Layle and daughter Alaina, thank you for supporting me through my many projects such as this book – I love you!

**M. Scott Echols, DVM, Dipl ABVP**

# TABLE OF CONTENTS

## CHAPTER 6
## HEMATOLOGY - THE WHITE BLOOD CELL COUNT AND IDENTIFICATION

## CHAPTER 7
## THE 3-H'S OF HEMATOLOGY

## CHAPTER 8
## COAGULATION TESTING

## CHAPTER 9
## MECHANICAL HEMATOLOGY

## CHAPTER 10
## ANTIGEN-ANTIBODY TESTING

## CHAPTER 11
## COPROPHOLOGICAL TESTING OF GASTROINTESTINAL FUNCTION

## CHAPTER 12
## MICROBIOLOGICAL PREPARATION

## CHAPTER 13
## MICROBIOLOGICAL SUPPLIES AND COLLECTION OF VETERINARY SPECIMENS

## CHAPTER 14
## MICROBIAL CULTURE AND SENSITIVITY AND BIOCHEMICAL TESTING

## CHAPTER 15
## MILK TESTING

## CHAPTER 16
## INTRODUCTION TO CYTOLOGY

## CHAPTER 17
## CYTOLOGY: THE ART OF FINE NEEDLE ASPIRATION

## CHAPTER 18
## NECROPSY: A TECHNICIAN'S ROLE

## CHAPTER 19
## AVIAN, EXOTIC MAMMALS, REPTILES AND FISH

# CHAPTER 20
# RUMEN FLUID COLLECTION AND EVALUATION

# APPENDICES

# INDEX

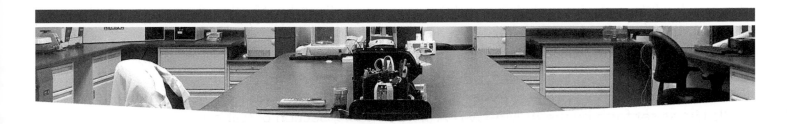

# CHAPTER 1

## THE CLINICAL PATHOLOGY LABORATORY

# OBJECTIVES

This lab introduces the student to the veterinary laboratory which is responsible for diagnostic testing as it relates to veterinary clinical pathology. Clinical laboratories may be individualized to fit the needs of the veterinary clinician and their expected clientele. Whether the needs include basic diagnostics for a rural large animal clinic, a cosmopolitan small animal practice or even a private state or federally run laboratory, many are the same.

This lab addresses the following Veterinary Technician Student Essential and Recommended Skills List as set forth by the AVMA-CVTEA in Appendix I, Section 6 - Laboratory Procedures. The Essential Decision-making Abilities to include:

✓ Properly prepare, handle and submit appropriate samples for diagnostic analysis in order to ensure maximum accuracy of results.
✓ Selection and maintenance of laboratory equipment.
✓ Implementation of quality control measures (group activity).

# KEY TERMS

Agglutination
Antigen-Antibody Reaction
Centrifuge
Culture and Sensitivity (C&S)
Cytology
Dermatophyte
Ectoparasite

Endoparasite
Fecal Floatation Solution
Hematology
Hemoglobinometer
Necropsy
Petri Dish
Point of Care Testing (POCT)

Refractometer
Reportable Disease
Sedi-Stain®
Urinalysis
Urinometer
Zoonotics

# LAB 1
# THE CLINICAL PATHOLOGY LABORATORY

# INTRODUCTION

There are many types of veterinary clinical pathology laboratories. As a student of veterinary technology, you are currently most interested in the academic laboratory which is associated with your studies and this course. It is important to realize that there are a variety of laboratories dedicated to veterinary clinical medicine that may prove to be viable future career opportunities for you upon graduation. Below is a brief summary of the most commonly seen veterinary laboratory situations.

## Discussion

The American Veterinary Medical Association – Committee on Veterinary Technician Education and Activities (AVMA-CVTEA) provides a concise and yet all-inclusive listing entitled: Veterinary Technology Student Essential and Recommended Skills List. This is a valuable resource both for the educator and the student; for the student this document allows a glimpse into all of the skills that make up a well-rounded veterinary technician once mastered. The list also allows students to understand the knowledge and skills that they must acquire before sitting for the Veterinary Technician National Examination (VTNE). Although there is no practical session to the VTNE, Section 4 pertains to laboratory procedures; a discipline that should be understood both didactically and practically.

The AVMA-CVTEA document may be found at: 'https://www.avma.org/education/center-for-veter-inary-accreditation/committee-veterinary-technician-education-activities/cvtea-accreditation-pol-icies-and-procedures-standards. Laboratory procedures are listed in Appendix I, No. 6 of the document and cover specimen management and sample analysis of urine, blood, ectoparasites, endoparasites, fecal material, cytology, and necropsy **(Figure 1-1)**. There are many types of material and equipment necessary for successful analysis of biological specimens. For the student's conve-nience, a proficiency check-off sheet is located in Appendix A. Students may wish to utilize this document to keep track of their progress in becoming proficient in each area of the AVMA-CVTEA Laboratory Procedures. Your instructor may wish to modify this listing if for instance Parasitology is taught as a stand-alone course at your institution.

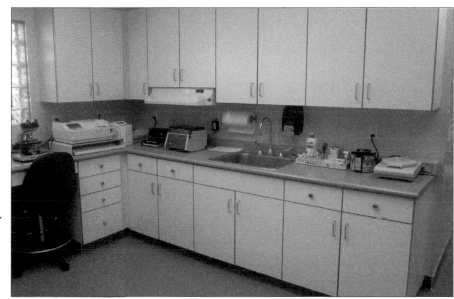

Figure 1-1: The veterinary clinical labora-tory is often filled with numerous useful diagnostics. Veterinary technicians often work within, or even manage, these types of laboratories.

# Types of Laboratories
## Clinical Veterinary Practice:

The veterinary practice which serves large, small or exotic animals will generally have the ability to complete basic laboratory procedures such as fecal examination (endoparasites, blood, fecal fat, etc.), urinalysis, hematology, and "basic ectoparasitic exams" including skin scrapings and identification. Typically a small amount of space is designated for these activities, often with point-of-care testing (POCT) being offered within the exam rooms **(Figure 1-2A-E)**. Clinical animal hospital labs are not normally certified or regulated in any special way. It is however possible to obtain certification through such organizations as the Veterinary Laboratory Association (VLA). Information on this organization may be found at http://www.vetlabassoc.com/ as well as more generalized hospital certification from American Animal Hospital Association (AAHA) to be found at https://www.aaha.org/.

## Academic Laboratory:

The academic setting such as you are currently working within as you complete this course may offer a variety of equipment including multiple types that essentially have the same function. Academic programs will often have more than one type of machine available for use. This serves a number of functions including: a) providing backup equipment in the event of malfunction, b) to expose students to various ways to accomplish clinical testing and c) expose students to both manual and mechanical testing methods, creating a well-rounded technician who can perform in any clinical situation. These labs are not required to be specially licensed or certified **(Figure 1-3)**.

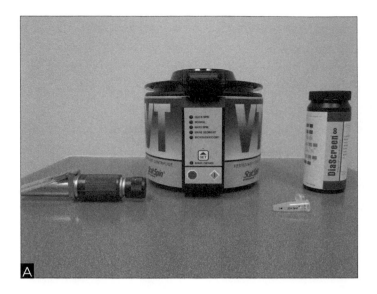

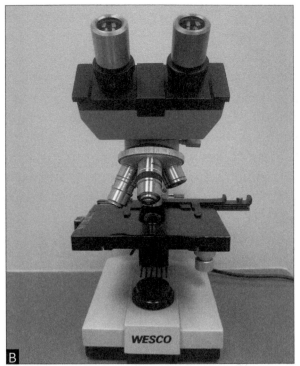

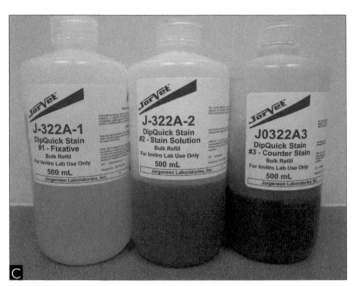

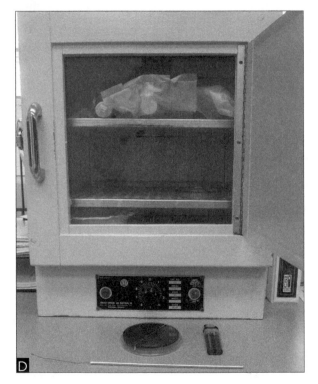

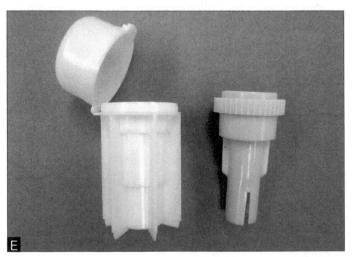

Figure 1-2A-E: Most clinical veterinary hospitals will have point of care equipment that allows the care team to perform quick diagnostic tests and provide answers while the animal is in the hospital. A refractometer, centrifuge, sample collection tubes and urine test strips are common in clinical practices (A). One of the most important diagnostic instruments in a veterinary practice is the microscope (B). In house stains such as those used for the 'Dip-Quick' method are also common (C). In-house microbiology stations are less commonly seen in private practice but can be very useful (D). Fecal parasite ova floatation equipment is a low cost and routine diagnostic test (E).

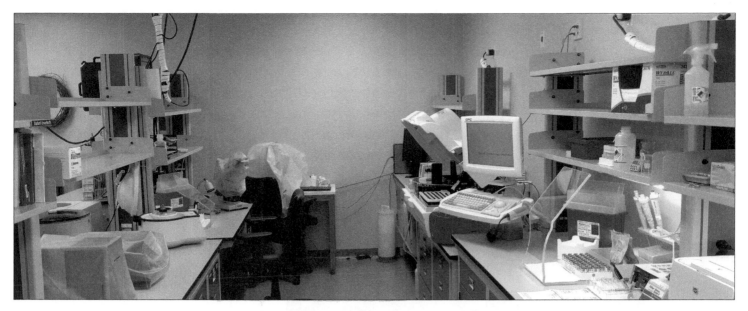

Figure 1-3: The academic laboratory can be very different from that of clinical practice and may include very specialized equipment to meet the needs of different studies in addition to more traditional diagnostics. This academic lab at North Carolina State University College of Veterinary Medicine carries equipment found in both traditional and specialty practices.

## Federal and State Laboratories:

Laboratories which offer agricultural and veterinary clinical testing and are part of either federal or state jurisdiction often fall under the auspices of the United States Department of Agriculture (USDA) or state Department of Agriculture. While these laboratories are equipped and staffed to perform any number of clinical testing procedures, they often dedicate a significant portion of their clinical resources to testing of samples that are suspected of being positive for any of the "reportable diseases" that are recognized by the National Animal Health Reporting System (NAHRS). Appendix B is a list of the 132 reportable diseases as of 2011. As government run laboratories, these labs are non-profit with a mission that is tied to both public health (i.e. zoonoses) and agricultural monitoring of veterinary medical concerns, particularly of the food animal industry **(Figure 1-4)**.

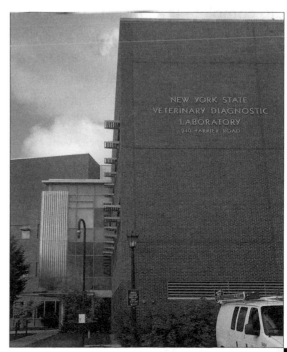

Figure 1-4: Federal and state laboratories must be prepared to test for infectious (including reportable) diseases along with other disease problems commonly encountered by their client base. As such, their equipment, testing methodologies, sample handling protocols and personnel guidelines can be quite specialized. Photo courtesy of Dr. Melissa King-Smith.

## Commercial Veterinary Laboratories:

Laboratories for veterinary medical research such as those operated by Pfizer, IDEXX and Hills Nutrition are often focused on research projects that correlate with the company interest and mission. For instance, laboratories associated with Hills Nutrition or IAMS would most likely be focused on nutritional research and development as it pertains to maintenance of canine and feline health. Pfizer or Merial laboratories may be focused more on the research and development of vaccines, fecal float solution, parasiticides and a variety of other veterinary pharmaceuticals **(Figure 1-5)**.

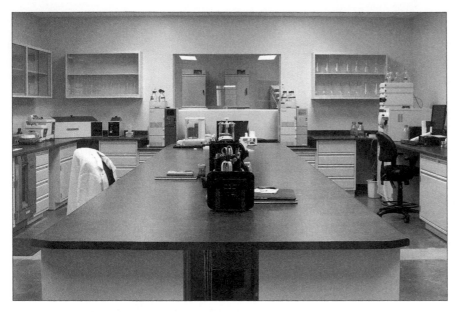

Figure 1-5: Commercial veterinary laboratories may include machines that can handle large sample volumes and specialized equipment for research purposes. Photo courtesy of Analytical Resource Labs, LLC, Lehi, UT.

# LABORATORY SESSION

The clinical pathology laboratory found in a typical veterinary technician program will be stocked with the equipment, supplies and reagents that are necessary to become proficient in the skills listed within the AVMA-CVTEA Essential Tasks and Skills List. Below is a list of supplies that students can expect to see in relation to skills which will be introduced and practiced to proficiency.

To complete the laboratory assignment for this lesson, students should perform an inspection of the lab based on the listing below. How many of the supplies and equipment listed does your lab possess? List the items and any supplies necessary to complete testing including mechanical equipment, disposable items and supplies that may not be on the list. Also indicate in your list, which equipment requires periodic maintenance and quality control, the time frame in which this is expected (i.e., daily, weekly, monthly, quarterly, etc.) and the person responsible. Throughout the course of the term, you will be learning the appropriate ways to perform quality control and in-house maintenance on the equipment which you use. Although students are encouraged to be creative when formatting this list, the following example is provided to illustrate the information that is required.

Refractometer:
| | |
|---|---|
| Uses: | Total Protein (serum/plasma) |
| | Specific Gravity (urine) |
| Supplies: | Microhematocrit Tubes |
| | Microcentrifuge |
| | Disposable Pipettes |
| | Lens Paper |
| Maintenance: | Daily cleaning of instrument is advised after each use |
| | Weekly calibration if used less than once daily |
| | Daily calibration if used daily |

Utilize the AVMA-CVTEA list to supplement your research and to answer the following questions:

1.  Does your laboratory facility have all of the necessary tools to complete your educational pursuit and clinical attainment of the skills listed in the AVMA-CVTEA list?

2.  If your facility lacks some of the equipment, what plan does the institution have for creating a learning environment to attain the skills?  Be specific in your answer?

# Equipment and Supplies for Specific Task Analysis
## Urinalysis: Manual Examination:
✓ Refractometer (specific gravity)
✓ Urinometer (specific gravity)
✓ Chemical test strips (may be used with Mechanical Urine Reader or manually)
✓ Sedi-Stain® (sedimentation testing)
  • Microscope
  • Test tubes
  • Slides and cover slips
✓ Physical properties (color, clarity, pH, odor)

## Mechanical Examination:
✓ UA Reader (IDEXX)

## Hematology: Manual Examination:
✓ Hemoglobinometer (Hgb)
✓ Hematocrit card (Hct)
✓ Refractometer (total protein of serum or plasma)
✓ Unopette reagent system
  • White blood count (WBC)
  • Red blood count (RBC)
  • Platelets
  • Reticulocytes
✓ Microscopes, slides and cover slips
✓ Microhematocrit tubes (PCV, fibrinogen)

## Mechanical Testing:
✓ Blood chemistry machines (IDEXX, Abaxis, etc.)

## Serology and Blood Parasite Examination: Manual Examination:
✓ Antigen-Antibody testing
✓ ELISA
✓ Slide card agglutination studies
✓ Knott's Filter Test
✓ Antigen-Antibody testing
 • Heartworm
 • Ehrlichia
 • *Borellia burgdorferi*
 • Others
✓ Mechanical testing (Heartworm: Abaxis)
✓ Microscope, slides and cover slips (manual direct examination of blood)

## Microbiological Studies:
✓ Petri dishes (cultures)
✓ Microscopes, slides and cover slips
✓ Sensitivity discs (culture and sensitivity)
✓ Media and reagents (pathogenic identification)
✓ California Mastitis Test (kit and reagents)
✓ Stains
 • Gram
 • Dip-Quick®
 • Negative
 • Phenol Cotton Blue (fungal)

## Cytology:
✓ Microscopes, slides and cover slips
✓ Staining sets (Dip-Quick® 3-part differential stain)
✓ Semen stain (Live-Dead Semen Stain)

## Necropsy:
✓ Set of necropsy instruments
✓ Culture jars and sampling containers (formalin, etc.)
✓ Swabs, forceps and syringes
✓ Carcass disposal bags

# REFERENCES

AVMA-CVTEA: Veterinary Technology Student Essential and Recommended Skills List. Accessed from: https://www.avma.org/education/center-for-veterinary-accreditation/committee-veterinary-technician-education-activities/cvtea-accreditation-policies-and-procedures-appendix-h

2011 National Animal Health Reporting System Reportable Disease List. Accessed from: http://www.aphis.usda.gov/animal_health/nahrs/downloads/2011_nahrs_dz_list.pdf

Fernandez, PJ; White, WR (2010) Atlas of Transboundary Animal Diseases. World Organization for Animal Health, Paris, France.

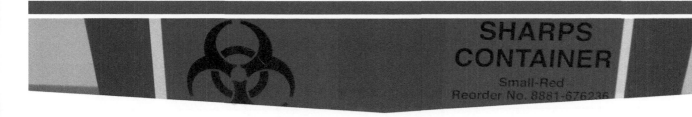

# CHAPTER 2

## LABORATORY AND ZOONOTIC SAFETY AND SANITATION

# OBJECTIVES

As a follow-up to the previous Introduction to the Clinical Pathology Lab, this lab introduces students to laboratory safety concerns as they pertain not only to laboratory activities but also the handling of animals during sample collection and the potential for zoonotic transmission. Veterinary technicians are not only at risk for accidental injuries such as punctures from medical sharps but also injury and zoonotic disease transmission due to contact with biological specimens as well as animal bites and scratches, or slips and falls sustained during collection. Students will learn precautionary measures that can be taken to prevent such occurrences from happening.

This lab addresses the following Veterinary Technician Student Essential and Recommended Skills List as set forth by AVMA-CVTEA in Appendix I, Section 1 – Office and Hospital Procedures, Client Relations and Communications.

✓ Maintain appropriate disposal protocol for hazardous materials.
✓ Establish and maintain appropriate sanitation and infection control protocols for a veterinary facility including patient and lab areas.

Appendix I, Section 6 – Laboratory Procedures.
✓ Understand how to ensure safety of patients, clients and staff.

# KEY TERMS

| | | |
|---|---|---|
| Cleaning | Medical Wastes | Right-to-Know |
| Disinfectant | MSDS | Sterilization |
| Ergonomic Injury | OSHA | Zoonotic Disease |
| Hazardous Materials | PPE | |

# LAB 2
# LABORATORY AND ZOONOTIC SAFETY AND SANITATION

# INTRODUCTION

The veterinary laboratory is full of opportunities for technicians to experience injury, disease transmission and in rare cases death. Because of the nature of veterinary clientele, it is possible to be injured during collection, testing or provision of care. For this reason, it is important for the veterinary technician to understand and recognize situations which may be problematic and act accordingly.

## Discussion

According to the AVMA-CVTEA guidelines, entitled Veterinary Technology Student Essential and Recommended Skills List, section 6: Laboratory Procedures – the veterinary technician must be fully capable of implementing the following guidelines for laboratory safety, sanitation and zoonotic concerns:

✓ Ensure safety of patients, clients and other staff.
✓ Properly prepare, label, package and store samples for laboratory analysis.

The directives address all actions from the time the decision is made to secure a sample until the animal is returned to the owner or cage at the completion of clinical sampling. Because the veterinary technician is often charged with collection as well as sample testing, they are placed at the helm of organizing and safely implementing such activities.

It should be noted that the animal is not the only source of concern in regard to laboratory safety. The laboratory itself hosts several "mini-environments" where injury may occur. **(Figure 2-1)** Some of these environments are discussed below however every lab is different and the laboratory within your clinic may have additional hazardous areas not mentioned in the context of this assignment. These areas should be examined, and appropriate safety measures discussed.

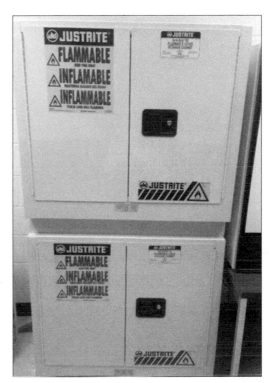

Figure 2-1: Hazards may be found throughout veterinary laboratories It is critical that the veterinary technician become aware of real and potential hazards such as may be stored in this well-marked chemical cabinet. An informed technician is better prepared to handle an emergency with hazardous materials than one not familiar with their surroundings.

# Physical Dangers – Fire

The possibility of a lab fire is an ever-present concern, not only as an accidental occurrence but also due to the amount of volatile substances and accelerants present within a pathology laboratory. Successful extinguishment of a fire is dependent on the type of fire encountered and therefore the "fuel" that allows the fire to burn. It is possible to accelerate a fire's destructive properties if the wrong type of extinguisher is used.

All fire extinguishers are not created equal. There are six common substances which may be used to extinguish a fire; they are water, foam spray, carbon dioxide, ABC powder, BC powder and D powder. Extinguishers are classified as A, B, C, D and K **(Table 2-1), (Table 2-2), (Figure 2-2)**.

## TABLE 2-1
## Fire Extinguisher Classifications

| CLASS | USAGE |
|-------|-------|
| A | Combustibles such as wood and paper |
| B | Flammable liquids (i.e. gas, oil) |
| C | Live electricity |
| D | Combustible metals |
| K | Combustible vegetable and animal oils and fats |

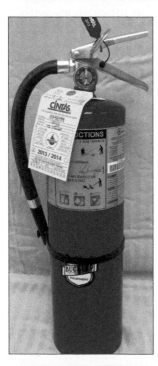

Figure 2-2: The 'A B C' type fire extinguisher is most commonly used in veterinary settings and is most appropriate for wood and paper combustibles, flammable liquids and electrical equipment.

## TABLE 2-2
## Fire Extinguisher Use

| EXTINGUISHER SUBSTANCE | PROPER USE | IMPROPER USE |
|-------------------------|------------|--------------|
| Water (H$_2$O) | Wood, paper, textiles | Live electrical equipment, flammable liquids, gaseous fires, flammable metal fires |
| Foam Spray (organic solvents, lauryl alcohol, corrosive inhibitors) | Wood, paper, textiles, flammable liquids | Live electrical fires, gaseous fires, flammable metal fires |
| Carbon Dioxide | Flammable liquids, live electrical fires | Gaseous fires, wood, paper, textiles, flammable metal fires |
| ABC Powder (mono-ammonium phosphate) | Wood, paper, textiles, flammable liquids, gaseous fires, live electrical fires | Flammable metal fires |
| BC Powder (sodium bicarbonate, potassium bicarbonate) | Flammable liquids, gaseous fires, live electrical equipment | Wood, paper, textiles, flammable metal fires |
| D Powder (graphite powder, sodium chloride granules) | Alkaline metal fires | Wood, paper, textiles, flammable liquids, gaseous fires |

Each area of the clinic should have the appropriate type of extinguisher handy for quick use. The acronym PASS reminds users of the sequence of operating a fire extinguisher safely and efficiently (regardless of type or class). Box 1 defines PASS more fully.

---

**BOX 1 USE OF FIRE EXTINGUISHER: PASS**
**P**: Pull the pin;
**A**: Aim the nozzle at the fire;
**S**: Squeeze the handle;
**S**: Sweep from side to side to put out flames.

---

# Physical Dangers - Chemical Injury

The clinical pathology laboratory setting is stocked with many different chemicals that have the potential for injury. These include burns (dermatological), splashes (eyes), accidental ingestion or inhalation (nose, mouth, throat), or accidental spills that may result in slips and falls (the number one reported injury in the workplace). It is essential to recognize these dangers before they happen and take precautions. While not exhaustive, **Table 2-3** lists common chemicals that are found in veterinary clinical lab settings and some of the dangers that they pose to personnel.

There are many types of "sharps" which may cause injury as a result of misuse or as a simple accident. Sharp items one may encounter in the lab include, needles, scalpels, broken glass, lancets and scissors or other bladed instruments to name a few. Many of these items are disposable; as a result, the possibility of injury during lab clean-up is reduced as they are discarded after use. Each laboratory should have a policy for disposal of such items **(Figures 2-3A&B)**.

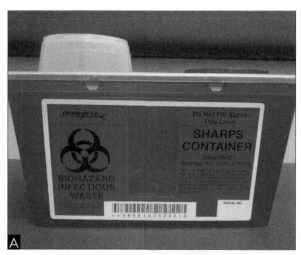
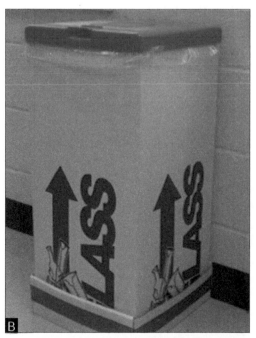

Figure 2-3A-B: 'Sharps' include anything that can puncture or cut human or animal tissue and generally implies small items such as needles and scalpel blades. Most small disposable sharps are placed in a 'Sharps Container' **(A)** while larger items such as broken glass are placed in other appropriate receptacles **(B)**.

# Zoonotics in the Lab

Because of the patient's ability to transmit diseases to veterinary personnel (i.e. zoonotic disease) through bites and scratches, laboratory personnel must guard against potentially life-threatening exposure. Exposure may occur at any time however there are three instances during which the risk of exposure is at its highest. They are:

    a) During restraint and handling of a veterinary patient
    b) During collection of samples
    c) During examination and testing of a sample

Exposure or infection may occur due to a bite or scratch, and also as a result of bodily fluid contamination (i.e. saliva, urine, feces) from a struggling animal (a). It is also possible to be "inoculated" with pathogenic substances through accidental needle sticks during blood draws or injections (b). The collection of samples from wounds and other exudates offers the opportunity for accidental ingestion or inhalation of infectious airborne particles or agents (c). Finally, the duties of a technician as carried out within the laboratory environment place them at risk of exposure as they handle samples that may more often than not come from sick animals (d). For this reason, it is imperative to recognize good lab practices and remain vigilant as to the need for lab safety during testing activities.

# Use of Personal Protective Equipment (PPE's)

The technician that works within a laboratory setting should make use of all personal protective equipment that is available as a way of ensuring that contamination and exposure to pathogens is kept at a minimum. Such items include gloves, masks, disposable aprons and a non-disposable, designated lab coat to wear within the lab **(Figure 2-4)**. This non-disposable item should be laundered weekly if not more often at the clinic and never taken home to be laundered with household items. All disposable items should be removed and discarded in the appropriate receptacle before exiting the lab to prevent spread of disease throughout other areas of the clinic.

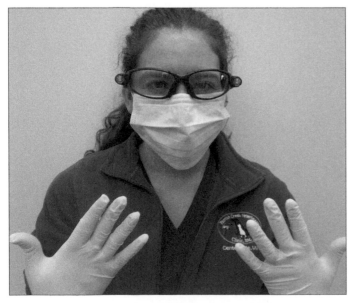

**Figure 2-4:** Personal protective equipment may include a mask, glasses and gloves (featured here) as well as an apron, N95 respirator and more depending on the need.

# LABORATORY SESSION – LABORATORY AND ZOONOTIC SAFETY AND SANITATION

The clinical pathology laboratory of a typical veterinary technician program will be enhanced with a variety of safety equipment, protocols and practices put into place for the safety of students, staff and the animals that they serve. It is important that those working and studying within this environment be familiar with the safeguards that are available in order to prevent accidents from happening. This lab assignment will serve to introduce the student to the features that are unique to each teaching lab.

## Lab Assignment – Chapter 2

This lab assignment is divided into two parts, both of which may be completed within a 2-hour lab session. For the first part of the lab, in order to complete the laboratory assignment for this lesson, students will act as laboratory detectives in a scenario that can only be described as troublesome and requires the sharp eye of someone familiar with good lab practices. Please refer to the page entitled "Bad Lab Assignment" for the scenario and instructions for completion. The second part of the lab involves a bit of "snooping around" within the laboratory in order to answer the following two multi-part questions. Please complete the lab, create a title page and staple all pages together to submit to your instructor.

1. What are the appropriate measures for disposal of the following items in the laboratory of your institution? Be concise in your answers.
    a. Needles, lancets
    b. Broken glass
    c. Used microscope slides and cover slips
    d. Tested and discarded urine and fecal samples
    e. Used tissues, paper and bench covers

2. Give a detailed explanation for how a dog and a cat should be safely restrained for the following procedures, including any equipment which can be used?
    a. Blood draw
    b. Fecal collection
    c. Urine collection via cystocentesis
    d. Skin scrapings from the top of the head
    e. Vaginal cytology sample using a Culturette® swab

# BAD LAB ASSIGNMENT

**THE STORY:**
**The pathology lab was assaulted by evil doers who do not respect lab safety and know nothing of prudent laboratory practices sometime during the night. Without disturbing anything, it is your job to inspect the lab and document below anything that may be unsafe or dangerous as well as just plain bad lab practice. There are at least 20 things wrong in this lab. Go find them.**

**Please do not disturb anything so everyone can have the same fun and chances to test their skills. Above all, have fun. Lab will be open to you and intact _____ (instructor will tell you days and times that lab will be open - fill in the blank with this information). Please complete your inspection during those hours. The lab will be discontinued after _____ (fill in with instructors directive).**

1. _____
2. _____
3. _____
4. _____
5. _____
6. _____
7. _____
8. _____
9. _____
10. _____
11. _____
12. _____
13. _____
14. _____
15. _____
16. _____
17. _____
18. _____
19. _____
20. _____

# REFERENCES

1. AVMA-CVTEA: Veterinary Technology Student Essential and Recommended Skills List. Accessed from: https://www.avma.org/education/center-for-veterinary-accreditation/committee-veterinary-technician-education-activities/cvtea-accreditation-policies-and-procedures-appendix-h
2. Hendrix, CM; Sirois, M; Laboratory Procedures for Veterinary Technicians, 5th Ed. St. Louis, Mosby-Elsevier, 2007.
3. Fire Extinguisher Solutions (website), Retrieved 9-6-2021 from: https://www.usfa.fema.gov/prevention/outreach/extinguishers.html

# CHAPTER 3

## URINALYSIS LABORATORY

## OBJECTIVES

This lab addresses the following Veterinary Technician Student Essential and Recommended Skills List as set forth by the AVMA-CVTEA in Appendix I, Section 6 – Laboratory Procedures.

✓ Properly package, handle and store specimens for laboratory analysis
✓ Prepare specimens for diagnostic analysis
✓ Select/maintain quality control of required lab equipment
✓ Determine physical properties (color, clarity, specific gravity)
✓ Test chemical properties
✓ Examine and identify sediment

## KEY TERMS

| | | |
|---|---|---|
| Bilirubin | Nitrites | Turbidity |
| Catheterization | Ova | Urates |
| Chloride | pH | Urea |
| Clarity | Phosphate | Uric Acid |
| Creatinine | Refractometer | Urine |
| Cystocentesis | Sediment | Urinometer |
| Ketones | Specific Gravity | Urobilinogen |
| Ketosis | Sulfate | |

# LAB 3
# URINE: THE COMPLETE ANALYSIS

## INTRODUCTION

Urine of domestic mammals is made up of approximately 96% water and 4% solid material. The solid matter is composed of urea, urates and uric acid as well as chloride, phosphates, sulfates and creatinine. The amount of urine which a normal dog or cat excretes daily varies although it is generally estimated to be approximately 20-40 mLs of urine per kilogram of body weight. Veterinary technicians are often called upon to collect and test urine samples within the clinical setting. Typically, samples are collected in one of the following manners as depicted in **Figure 3-1A-E**.

The choice of collection method may rely on two factors: the reason for testing and the type of sample required. If you are performing a routine urinalysis as part of a yearly wellness exam, the results of a manual collection will suffice, however if the objective is to collect a specimen for a bacterial culture and sensitivity, you will be better served with urine collected by either catheterization or cystocentesis to avoid outside contamination.

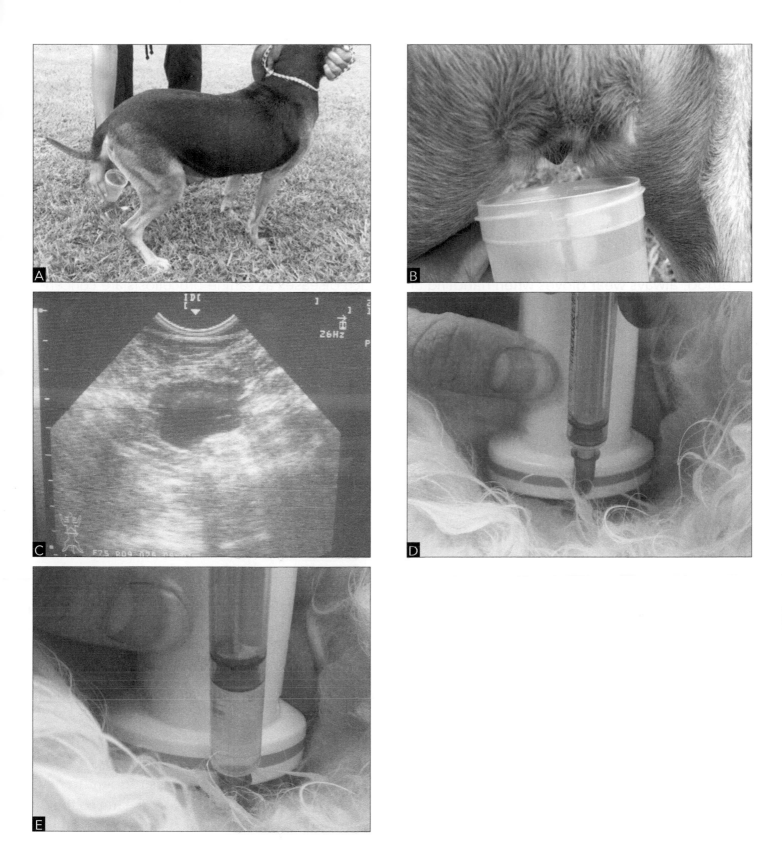

Figure 3-1A-E: Urine is typically collected by one of several means in domestic animals. The least sterile method is to simply collect fresh urine from a non-porous surface by aspirating with a sterile syringe. With a 'free catch' the animal is generally walked outside, and a clean plastic container is held (by hand or via an extension device) under the vulva or tip of the penis (A-B). The urethra (easily identified in males and difficult in females) can be catheterized and urine is collected straight from the urinary bladder. Ultrasound guided cystocentesis involves using an ultrasound (C) to identify the urinary bladder and then inserting a sterile needle through the body wall (usually caudal ventral abdomen) (D) and collecting the urine (E). With practice, cystocentesis can be performed without an ultrasound guide. These methods are listed from the least to most sterile urine collection methods.

# DISCUSSION
## Sample Collection and Storage
Regardless of the collection method, if urine is not handled correctly, it will begin to degrade rapidly, the pH will change, cellular alteration and bacterial overgrowth may occur. For this reason, if the sample is not to be tested immediately, it should be sealed and placed in a refrigerator (chilled, not frozen); the reduction in temperature will aid in preservation and slow growth of present bacteria.

When collected, the preferred method of storage is a plastic container with a threaded lid or a plain, sealed test tube **(Figure 3-2A&B)**. The lid should always be tightly secured to avoid contamination or leakage. Exam gloves should be worn during collection regardless of the collection method; always wear gloves when handling urine. Such diseases as canine brucellosis are concentrated in male canine urine while *Brucella abortus* can cause zoonotic diseases in humans.

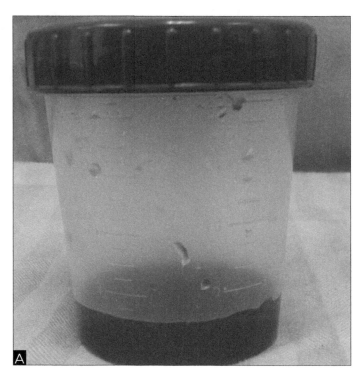 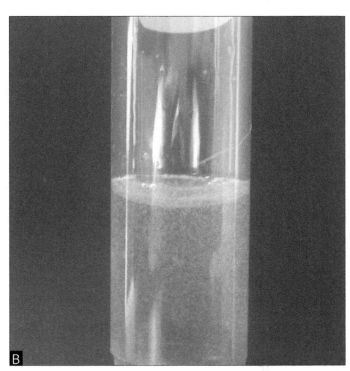

Figure 3-2A-B: Urine should be stored in a plastic container with a threaded lid (A) or a plain, sealed test tube (B).

## Shipping and Handling
Urine samples must sometimes be sent to an outside laboratory facility. It is always prudent to have at least three layers of protection between the sample and the courier/postal worker. Due to the frequent changes in postal regulations, refer to the following website: www.usps.com for updates by searching for "Biological Substances category B". For common couriers such as United Parcel Service and Federal Express, consult their webpage instructions which are updated regularly.

An example of proper packaging might include collecting the sample in a plastic cup with a tightened threaded lid (protective layer #1), place the cup in a zip lock bag that is sealable (protective layer #2), then place the sample in a cardboard box (protective layer #3) and pack either newspaper, paper towels or Styrofoam popcorn around the sample (protective later #4) before sealing and labeling. In addition to legible sent to and sent from addresses, always mark the box with the words "Biological Specimen" prominently displayed.

# LABORATORY SESSION – URINALYSIS

To complete each type of testing method, each student should have a total volume of 10 mL of fresh animal urine.

## Student Supplies

- ✓ 10 mL of fresh urine in a sealed urine cup
- ✓ Graduated cylinder (50 mL)
- ✓ Paper with text
- ✓ Refractometer **(Figure 3-3)**
- ✓ Urinometer **(Figure 3-4)**
- ✓ Urine chemistry strips **(Figure 3-5)**
- ✓ Microscope slide/cover slip **(Figure 3-6)**
- ✓ Microscope
- ✓ 15mL conical tube (2)
- ✓ Test tube and test tube rack
- ✓ Transfer pipette
- ✓ Sharpie marker
- ✓ Sedi-Stain®
- ✓ Urine culture set **(Figure 3-7)**

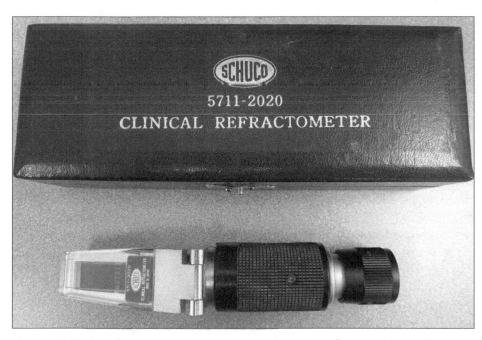

Figure 3-3: A refractometer measures urine specific gravity and mammalian plasma protein.

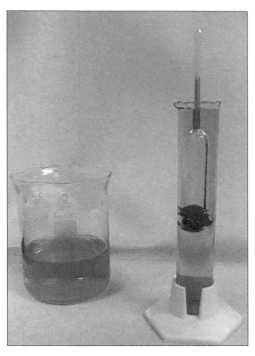

**Figure 3-4:** A urinometer is a simple instrument designed to measure urine specific gravity. Cow urine is in a beaker on the left and in the urinometer on the right. Picture Courtesy of Holly Thomas.

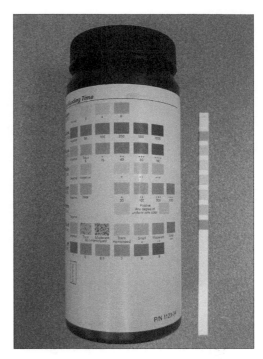

**Figure 3-5:** Numerous urine chemistry strips are available for domestic mammals. These easy to use strips give color coded values for a variety of urine chemistries including pH, glucose and more.

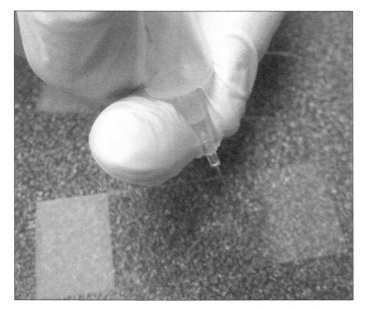

**Figure 3-6:** Clean microscope slides and coverslips (not shown here) are vital when collecting tissue or fluid samples. Here sediment from a spun urine sample is collected in a syringe and gently placed on to a clean slide for microscopic analysis.

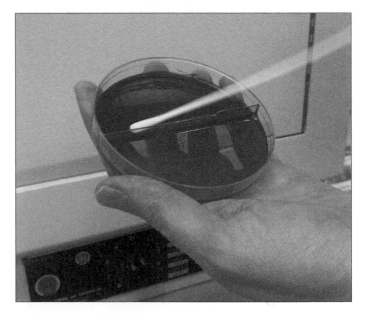

**Figure 3-7:** Culture of urine samples is commonly performed. Here a blood agar split with MacConkey agar plate is streaked with centrifuged urine sediment for in-house cultures.

# Classroom Supplies (to be shared)
✓ Centrifuge **(Figure 3-8)**
✓ Automatic urine reader

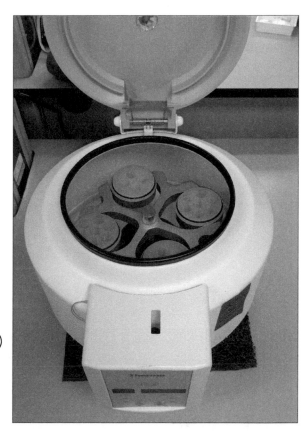

**Figure 3-8:** Centrifuges are all designed to separate different density particles into layers within a fluid sample. With urine, centrifuges generally separate the supernatant (top liquid portion) from the sediment (bottom more solid portion). The sediment often contains cells, crystals and other solid components commonly found in urine. The picture shows a swinging bucket type centrifuge. Picture courtesy of Holly Thomas.

# TEST: Physical Characteristics

Physical characteristics include assessing volume, color, clarity and odor. The volume of the urine specimen may be measured by a graduated cylinder; also, many urine collection cups have etched measurements on the outside surface of the cup for easy viewing. This information and urine color should be noted on the urine results form. **Table 3-1** indicates color variations and the possible significance.

| TABLE 3-1<br>Urine Color ||
| --- | --- |
| **URINE COLOR** | **POSSIBLE SIGNIFICANCE** |
| Pale Yellow | ↓ Urine concentration<br>↓ Specific Gravity<br>↑ Hydration |
| Medium Yellow | ↑ Specific Gravity<br>↓ Urine Output (oliguria)<br>↓ Hydration |
| Yellow | Normal Urine |
| Greenish/Brown | Presence of Bile |
| Reddish/Brown | Presence of blood/blood products |
| Orange | Drug Therapies |

It should be noted that some animal species produce urine in seemingly abnormal shades and colors. The rabbit typically excretes urine that is turbid (i.e. cloudy) with colors which may range from light yellow to reddish brown (often mistaken for blood and is due to porphyrin pigments and crystaluria). The following pictures show the contrast in colors of normal dog, rabbit, horse and cow urine as collected by manual methods **(Figure 3-9 A–E)**.

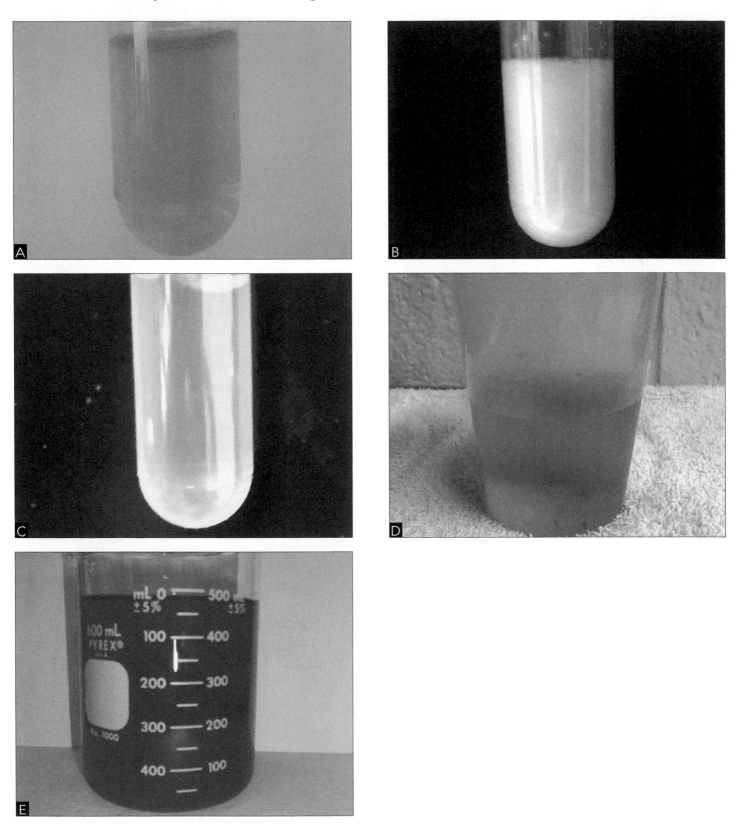

**Figure 3-9A-E:** Normal urine can vary in appearance between species and it is important to understand these differences prior to making interpretations. Normal dog urine is slightly straw colored and should have no to minimal visible sediment (A). However, rabbits and guinea pigs may normally have a large (B) or minimal (C) amount of sediment which is largely related to the rabbit's or guinea pig's diet. Cow urine is normally fairly clear (Photo courtesy of Melissa King-Smith) (D). Normal horse urine (E).

The normal clarity or transparency of urine is clear, however there are exceptions. The rabbit and the female horse normally excrete urine that is somewhat turbid. When recording transparency readings of a urine specimen the following terms are commonly used to describe the level of clarity: clear, slight cloudiness, cloudy or turbid. Placing a page with text behind the specimen in order to gauge clarity is helpful and the following results are relevant descriptions (**Figure 3-10**):

✓ Easily read letters = clear
✓ Slight distortion of letters, can still read = slight cloudiness
✓ Major distortion of letters, letters hard to see = cloudy
✓ No letters visible = turbid

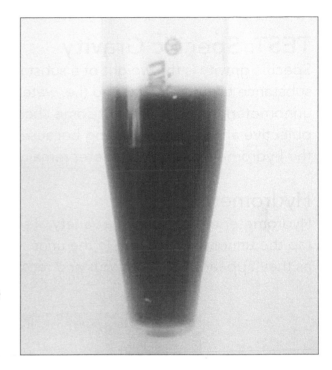

Figure 3-10: By placing a piece of white paper behind the urine sample the urine color may be more easily described. Written words on the paper can also help define clarity of the sample. The more difficult the letters are to read through the urine, the more turbid the sample. Bloody (red tinged) dog urine is shown here.

The cloudiness of rabbit urine is a result of calcium carbonate excretion.

Equine urine is cloudy due to the amount of mucus normally present; this is a normal finding.

It is important to note that urine that is allowed to sit at room temperature for long periods of time will lose its clarity and therefore be misjudged in terms of diagnostic usefulness.

The final physical characteristic of urine is the odor. When checking the odor of any specimen or chemical in a laboratory setting, always utilize the wafting technique. This technique is performed by simply cupping your hand above the specimen or chemical container and wafting the air toward your face, while at the same time inhaling gently to avoid overwhelming your sensory organs. While odor does not indicate a great deal diagnostically, it can be useful especially if it is sweet or fruity smelling. This may be a sign of diabetes mellitus, bovine ketosis or ovine pregnancy disease.

## LAB EXERCISE

Pour the urine sample into the graduated cylinder and record the amount that you have on your results sheet. Now place the text page behind the urine to determine the clarity (transparency) and record on your results sheet. Proceed to the next step.

To test odor, utilize the wafting technique by placing the container of urine on the countertop and wafting the air towards your face, while gently sniffing until an odor is detected. Do not place your nose directly over the specimen container and inhale as this may contaminate the specimen and possibly the tester. Describe the odor on the lab results page. Some common choices are "normal", "fruity", "strong" or "ammonia".

To ascertain color, view the urine in a clear container under normal light conditions. Refer to Table 3-1 and enter your findings on the results sheet. You may find it helpful to place the container on a white piece of paper for best results.

# TEST: Specific Gravity

Specific gravity is the weight of a substance compared with the weight of an equal amount of some substance taken as a standard (i.e. water). This may be measured by utilizing a hydrometer (i.e., urinometer), refractometer or some chemistry reagent strips. The refractometer provides a more objective and accurate reading because it can be calibrated and requires significantly less urine than the hydrometer. The hydrometer remains useful in many practices as a less expensive alternative.

## Hydrometer:

Hydrometer tubes come in a variety of sizes. Fill the tube three quarters full with fresh urine. Gently tap the urinometer, place it in the urine and spin. When the spinning motion stops, read the results as they appear at the meniscus and record them on the lab results sheet **(Figure 3-11)**.

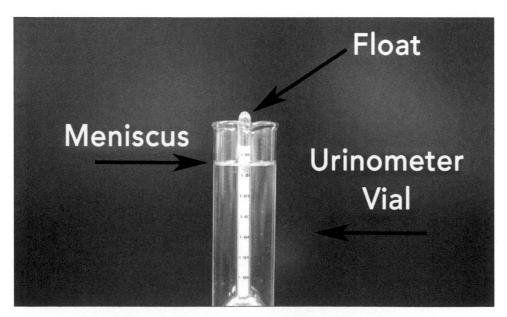

Figure 3-11: Series of steps describing use of a urinometer. 1. Calibrate the urinometer using distilled water which should read 1.0. Fill the urinometer two thirds full using room temperature distilled water. Gently lower the float into the water and impart a slight spin on the stem to keep it from sticking to the sides of the urinometer vial. Read the bottom of the meniscus once stabilized. Temperature adjustments will need to be made if not properly calibrated. 2. Following calibration, fill the urinometer vial two thirds full using the urine sample. Lower the float and spin as before. Read the bottom of the meniscus as before. Adjust the value read based on any calibration performed. If the urinometer reads 1.0 during distilled water calibration, no adjustment to the urine sample value is required. Picture courtesy of Austin Davis.

## Refractometer:

Place a drop of urine on the glass of the refractometer, close the plastic guard over the specimen and point it toward a light source. By rotating the eyepiece, focus on the "horizon" line and bring it into sharpness. Read the S.G. scale to ascertain the results before recording them on your lab results sheet. The refractometer is the preferred method of determining specific gravity because the instrument can be calibrated. Calibration of a refractometer is done by placing a drop of distilled water on the prism of the instrument and adjusting the scale to 1.000 which is the specific gravity of water. Record the results for both methods of obtaining specific gravity on the lab results sheet (See Figure 3-3).

## TEST: Urine Chemistries

The urine sample contains many chemical components found in varying amounts. The amount measured may be useful in diagnosing or determining homeostasis (Table 3-2).

| TABLE 3-2 Chemical Components Commonly Found In Urine | |
|---|---|
| **CHEMICAL** | **SIGNIFICANCE OF PRESENCE IN URINE SPECIMEN** |
| Bilirubin | Red blood cell destruction, liver disease, bile duct obstruction |
| Blood | Trauma, urinary tract Infection, inflammation of renal system |
| Glucose | Proximal tubule malabsorption decreased tubular re-sorption malfunction, diabetes mellitus |
| Ketones | Starvation, insulinoma, diabetic ketoacidosis, hypoglycemia, high fat, low carb diet, glycogen storage diseases |
| Leukocytes | Dogs: pyuria and other infectious processes, Cats: prostatitis (Beware of false negatives caused by antibiotic therapy or false positives caused by fecal contamination). |
| Nitrites | Bacterial infections |
| pH | Dietary changes (more meat), increased glucose, bacterial infection, exposure to air (post-collection) |
| Protein | Hemorrhage, renal disease, urinary tract infection |
| Specific Gravity | Increased S.G. = level of protein; Decreased S.G. = alkaline urine |
| Urobilinogen | Intestinal or liver malfunction |

## Reagent Strips:

Several different brands of chemical reagent strips are available for use in the measurement of the levels of chemical components found in urine (See Table 3-2). Even though there are several different brands available for purchase, all function in virtually the same way. In order to perform this test, urine is dropped onto the strip using a dropper or pipette. It is recommended not to "dip" the strip into the urine because this may lead to contamination of the sample and is messy. By pipetting the urine onto the individual pads of the strip, you effectively coat each piece of litmus paper on the strip. The strip is then taped to the side of the collection cup to remove excess urine. Results are read at immediate, 30 second and 60 second intervals (or as directed on the package). **Figure 3-12** shows two strips, the first has not been utilized while the second has been loaded with urine and is ready to read.

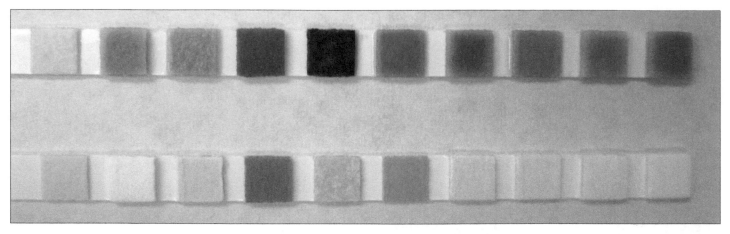

Figure 3-12: Urine chemistry reagent strips consist of a series of square chemical reagent pads on a plastic strip. Urine is placed in each chemical reagent pad (per manufacturer's instructions) and the strip is read after a set amount of time (usually 30 to 60 seconds). The bottom strip is clean. Bloody urine was applied to the top strip dramatically changing several of the values as indicated by the color differences.

## Automatic Urine Analyzer (Reader):

Automatic urine analyzers, commonly called "UA Readers" are available. The analyzer functions by analyzing urine soaked, chemical reagent strips and reporting/providing printed results. **Figure 3-13** shows an example of a loaded urine reader (IDEXX).

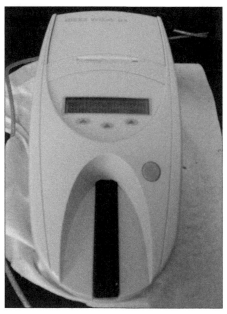

Figure 3-13: An automatic urine analyzer is a device that performs automated urine testing in a clinical setting. Such devices can often read urine chemistry strips and/or specific analytes such as bilirubin, glucose, red blood cells and protein.

# LAB EXERCISE

Complete this exercise if you have access to an automatic urine analyzer, if you do not have access, review the way in which the automatic urine analyzer works in your textbook in order to complete this exercise.

Utilizing the previously collected urine sample, do a comparison of the time needed to perform the test using the dip stick method and the automatic urine analyzer, and the results obtained. Record the dip stick results in the lab report.

# TEST: Microscopic Examination

With the exception of horse and rabbit urine, it is considered abnormal to find large amounts of sediment in the urine of domestic animal species. The presence and composition of urinary sediment within a specimen should be regarded as diagnostically significant.

To evaluate sediment place 10 mls of urine in a test tube, centrifuge the sample for five minutes (1000 to 2000 rpm's), and pour off the supernatant in one fluid motion. Add a drop of Sedi-Stain® and re-suspend the liquid by tapping on the side of tube to re-mix the sediment. Pipette a drop of urine onto a microscope slide and place a cover slip over the liquid. Examine the slide under a high power objective (40x), and identify the solid elements that are seen.

The study of urinary sediment is vast enough to fill whole chapters in textbooks. Among the findings you might expect to encounter are the following: erythrocytes, leukocytes, epithelial cells (renal tubular, transitional, and squamous), neoplastic cells, casts (fatty, waxy, granular), bacteria, yeasts/fungi, parasites and crystals (struvites, calcium carbonate, ammonium urate, calcium oxalates). **Table 3-3** provides a quick reference for the various casts and crystals which may be encountered while **Table 3-4** provides a quick reference guide for sediments.

| TABLE 3-3 Sediment Crystals | | |
| --- | --- | --- |
| **CRYSTALS** | **APPEARANCE** | **MEDICAL IMPLICATIONS** |
| Bilirubin | Yellow, reddish brown needles | Abnormal bilirubin metabolism |
| Calcium Oxalate | Squares | Ethylene glycol toxicity, hypercalciuric disorders |
| Calcium Phosphate | Yellow spheres, long prisms, colorless | Normal but can indicate calcium phosphate uroliths |
| Cystine | Hexagonal shape, colorless | Uroliths |
| Drug Induced* *Sulfonamide | Sheaves of needle shaped crystals | Drug therapy |
| *Radio-Opaque Solution | Colorless needles | Drug therapy |
| *Ampicillin | Long, thin needles or prisms | Drug therapy |
| Ammonia Urates | Brown/yellow thorny apple shape | Common uroliths formation in Dalmations & English Bulldogs |

## TABLE 3-4
## Various Urine Sediments

| SEDIMENT FINDING | ORIGIN/CAUSE | APPEARANCE | CELL TYPE | MEDICAL IMPLICATIONS |
|---|---|---|---|---|
| RBC | Hemorrhage | Anuclear disc, pale to colorless OR Anuclear disc pale to colorless | Erythrocyte | Strenuous exercise, trauma, stones, infection, neoplasms |
| WBC | Infection or inflammation | Spherical granulated single/clumps Frequent nucleus degeneration | Neutrophils Eosinophils Lymphocytes Monocytes | Pyuria Urinary Tract infection Inflammation |
| Epithelial Cells | Renal tubules | Round, central, spherical nucleus Granulated cytoplasm | Epithelial | Not a reliable indicator of health |
| Transitional Epith. Cells | Urothelium | Large, flat, spindle shaped, polygonal | Epithelial | Renal inflammation Cancer |
| Squamous Epith. Cells | Malignancy | Large, thin, plate like | Epithelial | Contaminated urine specimen Cancer |
| Neoplasms | Malignancy | Nucleus enlargement, structural changes, multinucleate aberrant forms | Epithelial | Carcinoma |
| Bacteria | UTI | Rods and cocci | Unicellular | Infections |
| Yeast/Fungi | Infections Contamination | Ovoid (Y) Filamentous (F) | Round (Y) Filament (F) | Contaminants Fungal cystitis |
| Parasites | Ova of *Dioctophyma renale*; *Capillaria plica*, *Chlamydophila felis/catis* Trophozoites | Oval, bipolar plugs, colorless, pitted shell Motile protozoa | Eggs of parasites Unicellular | Parasitic infection |

| CASTS TYPE | ORIGIN/CAUSE | APPEARANCE | MEDICAL IMPLICATIONS |
|---|---|---|---|
| Casts | Mucoprotein Formation of debris | Cylindrical | Minor pathological changes in renal tubule |
| Hyaline Cast | Glomerular capillary walls | Cylindrical | Mild-severe renal disease, proteinuria |
| Epithelial Cast Fatty Cast Granular Cast Waxy Cast | Tubular epithelial cells | Cylindrical | Degeneration/necrosis of epithelial tubular cells, infarction, nephro-toxins |

# QUICK REFERENCE GUIDE

## Specific Gravity

### Urinometer:
1. Fill urinometer tube ¾ full with urine.
2. Place hydrometer in tube and spin then tap.
3. Read at the bottom of the meniscus.

### Refractometer:
1. Fold open the plastic top of the refractometer.
2. Place a drop of urine on the glass prism.
3. Close top over the urine.
4. Hold refractometer up to artificial or natural light and look through eyepiece.
5. Read specific gravity at the horizontal mark.
6. Make sure you are reading the side that is marked S.G.
7. Wipe the prism clean with a water-moistened paper towel and dry after usage.

### Chemistries: Chemical Strip Tests:
1. Place a fresh strip on a paper towel flat on counter.
2. Using a dropper or pipette, place a drop of urine on each litmus square fully covering the square.
3. Tap strip on the side of the urine container to dislodge excess urine.
4. Read according to instructions, paying close attention to time.

Automatic Urine Reader: Please refer to the manufacturer instructions that accompany the machine.

### Microscopic Evaluation (Sediment):
1. Place 10 mLs of urine in a tube and centrifuge for 5 minutes at 1000 to 2000 rpm's.
2. Pour off the supernatant in one fluid motion.
3. Add one drop of Sedi-Stain and re-suspend the sediment by tapping on the tube to mix.
4. Pipette a sample of stained sediment onto a microscope slide and place a cover slip over the stained sample.
5. View under high power objective (4x) to identify sediment.

# URINALYSIS WORKSHEET

Due Date: _____

## Instructions

Based on what you have learned in the lab today, please answer the following questions. Your instructor may request that this worksheet be submitted to count as part of your lab grade.

## Scenario:

Zippy, a 5 year old intact male, cocker spaniel that weighs 28 pounds is brought in by his owner. The owner states that Zippy is drinking more than normal and urinating more frequently although it appears that he is producing small amounts of urine. Because the owner is a registered nurse, she has been monitoring Zippy's urine output for two days prior to coming to the clinic. She reports that on Monday Zippy urinated approximately 187 mLs and on Tuesday he urinated approximately 204 mLs. Using this case scenario and what you have learned in this lab, please answer the following questions.

1. Is the dog excreting a normal amount of urine daily for his weight? Explain._____
_____.

2. The veterinarian, Dr. Wormum would like a sterile urine sample from Zippy. What procedure should you set up for? List all supplies that are needed._____
_____
_____

3. The urine was collected at 9:45 this morning, Dr. Wormum would like for you to run a full urine panel in-house immediately. Based on what you know about physical characteristics and Zippy's history so far, what color would you expect the urine to be and why?_____
_____
_____

4. Dr. Wormum collected a total of 18 mLs of urine by the method discussed in # 2. Given the protocol for testing urine as discussed in this lab, do you have enough urine?_____
_____

5. The specific gravity reading was conducted on Zippy's urine twice, once with the refractometer and once using the urinometer/hydrometer set-up. The results were as follows: Refractometer: 1.026; Urinometer/hydrometer: 1.022. According to Blackwell's 5-Minute Veterinary Consult: Canine and Feline textbook, normal specific gravity is >1.030. Which reading is more reliable and less subjective and why; how do you interpret these results._____
_____

6. Based on the chemical reagent strips used in your lab, list the correct chemical reagent under the correct time lapse for ascertaining a correct and accurate reading/reporting of results.

| IMMEDIATE | 30 SECONDS | 60 SECONDS |
|---|---|---|
| | | |
| | | |
| | | |
| | | |
| | | |

7. Which species routinely has large amounts of sediment in the urine which is normally cloudy and may be reddish brown in color._____

_____

8. This species of animal typically has mucus within its urine, and this generally occurs in only one sex. Please list the species and the sex that this phenomenon is likely to occur in:_____

_____

[NOTE: Questions 9 and 10 are "challenge" questions which necessitate research outside of the lab manual to find the answers, this is necessary to cultivate good research skills in students].

9. What is the genus and species name for the New Zealand White rabbit, a common laboratory animal that produces turbid, reddish brown urine?_____

10. Hypercalcinuria is commonly called _____ and is defined as _____ _____ in rabbits.

# REFERENCES

1. Hendrix, C., & Sirois, M. (2007). Laboratory Procedures for Veterinary Technicians, 5th Ed. St. Louis, MO: Mosby-Elsevier.

2. JM Science. (2010, December 10). Smelling a Chemical: The Wafting Technique. Retrieved from Lab Manager Magazine: https://www.labmanager.com/lab-health-and-safety/smelling-a-chemical-the-wafting-technique-19098#:~:text=lapse%20in%20concentration.-,When%20you%20are%20in%20the%20laboratory%20and%20take%20a%20direct,the%20air%20toward%20your%20face.

3. Osborne, C., & Stevens, J. (1999). Urinalysis: A Clinical Guide to Compassionate Patient Care. Shawnee Mission, KS: Bayer Corporation.

4. Pressler, B. (2009). Cystocentesis. In J. S. S.L. Vaden, Blackwell's Five-Minute Veterinary Consult: Laboratory Tests and Diagnostic Procedures (pp. 202-204). Ames, IA: Wiley-Blackwell Publishing.

5. Sink, C., & Feldman, B. (2004). Urinalysis. In C. Sink, & B. Feldman, Laboratory Urinalysis and Hematology for the Small Animal Practitioner (pp. 3-44). Jackson, WY: Teton NewMedia.

6. Tartaglia, L., & Waugh, A. (2002). Attainment of Nutrients and Disposal of Wastes. In L. Tartaglia, & A. Waugh, Veterinary Physiology and Applied Anatomy (p. 128). Oxford, England: Butterworth-Heinemann Publishers.

7. Taylor, D., & V. Lee, D. M. (2010). Rabbits (Chapter 12). In B. Ballard, & R. Cheek, Exotic Animal Medicine for the Veterinary Technician, 2nd ed. (p. 282). Ames, IA: Wiley-Blackwell.

8. V.P. Studdert, C. G. (2012). Saunders Comprehensive Veterinary Dictionary, 4th Ed. St. Louis, MO: Saunders-Elsevier Publishing.

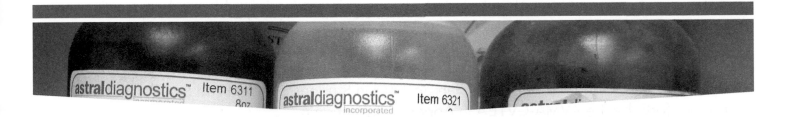

# CHAPTER 4

## PROPER LABORATORY TREATMENT OF BLOOD SMEARS AND CELLS

# OBJECTIVE

This lab introduces the student to the manner in which blood smears should be handled and some of the abnormalities that can occur as a result of mishandling of blood during the collection, creation and staining of smears. Although veterinary technicians do not (and should never) offer a diagnosis as a result of examining a blood smear, they should be knowledgeable about the normal and abnormal features that may be encountered in a blood smear and the possible reasons for these occurrences.

This lab addresses the following Veterinary Technician Student Essential and Recommended Skills List as set forth by the AVMA-CVTEA in Appendix I, Section 6:
- ✓ Evaluate erythrocyte morphology – normal vs. abnormal
- ✓ Perform leukocyte differential – normal vs. abnormal

# KEY TERMS

| | | |
|---|---|---|
| Adrenaline | Hemostasis | Phlebotomist |
| Artifacts | Homeostasis | Precipitate |
| Buccal Bleeding Time | Leukocytes | Safety Data Sheet |
| Crenation | Material Safety Data Sheet | SDS |
| Epinephrine | MSDS | Vacuoles |
| Erythrocytes | Mammal | Vasopressor |
| Glycogenesis | Nucleated Erythrocyte | |

# INTRODUCTION

The blood sample is made up of a variety of blood cell types all having their specific function and role to play in maintaining hemostasis. The cells are fragile and subject to damage which may be caused by pathologic damage, mishandling and even genetic disorders. Some cells differ "normally" based on the species of animal in which they are found. A prime example is the nucleated erythrocyte found in birds, reptiles and most fish which is absolutely normal for these species **(Figure 4-1)**. Nucleated erythrocytes in mammalian species, however, represent possible anemia and release of immature erythrocytes into the circulating blood, an abnormality to be recognized when examining the peripheral blood smear of any animal that is classified as a mammal.

## Discussion

The ability to recognize normal from abnormal within a blood smear rests to a great degree upon having a solid understanding of the process of creating a good blood smear, a task that begins with procuring a usable blood sample. There are many external factors that may influence the quality of the final product - the blood smear, and it is up to the technician to know, recognize and prevent as many of these factors from occurring as possible. For the purpose of self-evaluation, the following is a brief review of some of the external activities which may ultimately affect blood cell appearance on the slide.

## Struggling Animal:

A struggling animal is not only difficult to deal with, but their wild gyrations as people try to hold them creates problems for the phlebotomist who is essentially attempting to spear a moving target. As the animal continues to struggle, there are physiological changes occurring as a result of the "fight or flight" to include the release of epinephrine (i.e. adrenaline) which acts as a vasopressor to increase blood pressure and heart rate. This hormone also increases glycogenolysis and the release of glucose from the liver. These hormonal actions while not necessarily problematic to blood cell morphology may affect certain blood chemistries and the complete blood count if tested.

The struggling of the patient during blood draws will affect cell morphology if the needle is moving back and forth, sliding in and out of the vein causing trauma to tissue, and damaging blood cell structure (i.e. erythrocyte crenation). For this reason, cease restraint and allow the animal to calm down, then re-attempt perhaps with "less" restraint. Some suggestions for success include less people, noise, drama and action. Consider how much of a quality blood sample you truly need and use smaller volumes such as 2 to 3 mL tubes for whole blood or even a drop of blood directly from the needle onto a slide for smearing and staining purposes.

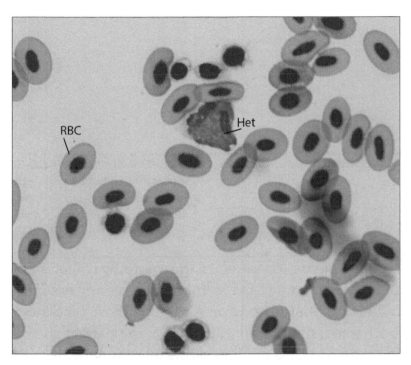

Figure 4-1: Nucleated red blood cells (RBC) are normal for fish, birds and reptiles but completely different from those found in normal mammals. Heterophils (Het) are also quite different between species. This blood smear comes from a bird.

## Blood Drawing Techniques:
Struggling animals aside, it is often difficult to draw blood due to such factors as small animals = small veins, anemia, illness, dehydration or venipuncture sites that are compromised due to burns, injury or loss of access. The technician must finesse their techniques as well as be creative in the procurement of the sample. It is often not possible to collect a larger sample; therefore, smaller amounts must be collected and divided up quickly. Consider how many tests may be completed using drops of blood as opposed to whole milliliters. While it may be less than ideal, a buccal bleeding test can be done in place of a PT or PTT in an emergency with a drop of blood, Whatman filter paper and a stopwatch with the results being supplied in just a few minutes. Likewise, a drop of blood placed in the glucometer (a point-of care [POC] testing device) can replace the full scale chemistry evaluation for a diabetic cat in crisis.

If a minute amount of blood is needed (as for a glucometer or to complete a packed cell volume) and the animal will not either tolerate blood loss (as with small animals and the severely anemic) or is fractious, consider collection via a 25 gauge needle or 1.0 cc or smaller syringe with a 27 g or smaller needle (such as an insulin syringe) **(Figure 4-2)**. Choose a vessel that results in the least amount of animal stress and insert a plain 25 gauge needle. As blood fills the needle hub, collect the blood using a hematocrit tube (micro-tube if needed) or POC testing strip or other device. Alternatively, use the small syringe and attached needle to collect just enough blood to complete the test. For those animals at risk of additional blood loss, ensure that hemostasis is adequate after the needle is removed.

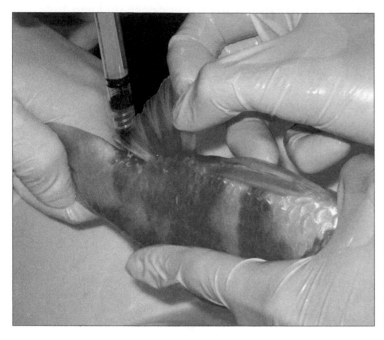

Figure 4-2: Proper restraint and equipment is essential to successful venipuncture. Just as an example of the potential variability encountered, blood is collected from the ventral tail vein of a properly and carefully restrained koi fish.

If blood must be collected in volume, consider using a butterfly catheter (23 to 26 gauge) to collect from small veins without undue trauma to the animal or the blood cells. There are several brands and configurations of butterfly catheter, however for the gentlest handling of blood, utilize the set which has a needle at both ends; the butterfly syringe for the patient and a needle for piercing the tube top. This avoids ruptured cells as blood flows into the tube. If butterfly catheters are not available and blood is drawn with a needle and syringe, do not squirt blood into the tube. It is better to remove the tube cap and needle from the syringe and allow blood to flow down the side of the tube walls until it is full **(Figure 4-3)**. Recap the tube and gently invert it to mix the blood with anticoagulant, never shake.

## Blood Storage:
Ideally blood should be analyzed as soon after drawing the sample as possible. If analysis occurs on blood left at room temperature for over 2 to 4 hours (depending on temperature) or after being refrigerated for more than 12 hours, artifacts may be seen. Certain white blood cells begin to degenerate with the nuclei and chromatin strands changing morphologically. These changes may appear as pathologic findings to the unsuspecting viewer or someone who is unfamiliar with the case history.

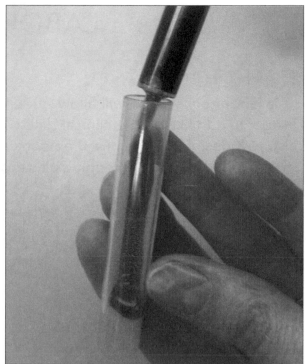

Figure 4-3: It is best to analyze blood immediately after collection. However, blood samples are often stored in appropriate containers for a short period after collection. For most stored blood samples, it is best to remove the top of the container and the needle from the syringe. Allow the blood to flow down the tube walls until full as opposed to forcefully squirting out the blood. The later can result in damage to the blood sample and erroneous results.

## Prep and Stain:

When preparing a peripheral blood smear, the blood must be handled carefully to avoid causing damage to the cells or the appearance of "pseudo-pathology". Blood smears which are stained prior to being completely dry can exhibit "drying pathology". These artifacts manifest themselves as erythrocytes which may be seen as any of the following: crescent shaped cells, areas that appear to be punched out, or exhibit the presence of vacuoles. It is also possible to improperly apply stain to a smear that is perfectly dry, resulting in artifacts or cellular mis-staining. For instance, when stain is not left on a slide long enough the nuclei of the leukocytes may be partly or completely unstained; this may also occur when the stain utilized is aged. Most commercial stains have an expiration date listed on the stock bottle, it is a good idea to treat this date the same as you do food at home for optimal usage. Likewise, when using secondary containers for stains (such as Coplin Jars) be sure to label the secondary containers with the expiration date as well as a Material Safety Data Sheet (MSDS) or Safety Data Sheet (SDS) label. The SDS has replaced the previously used MSDS method of labelling. It is possible, even in stains that are not past the expiration date, if used for "dirty" samples such as fecal, ear and abscess cytology for stains to become contaminated and useless. This may result in the appearance of bacteria, yeast, fungi and other organisms on future stains giving false positive results. It is best to have a 'dirty' and a 'clean' stain set that are used separately. The 'dirty' stain set will need to be changed more frequently due to contamination.

One final note regarding Wright's Stain, specifically: if stored for a lengthy period or left on slides for an extended period of time, a precipitate may form and adhere to the slide giving the appearance of a foreign body, hematological parasite or other abnormality. It is possible to strain the stain through Whatman filter paper to remove precipitate, but you should consider replacing the stain completely.

# LABORATORY SESSION

## INTRODUCTION

This laboratory session will allow students to investigate the stains that are available to them before usage. In addition to the clinical skills which technicians need to hone, the technician is generally also responsible for the procurement and maintenance of laboratory supplies to include monitoring of expiration dates and keeping all supplies current.

## MATERIAL AND SUPPLIES LIST

| | | |
|---|---|---|
| Aprons/lab coats | Gloves | Stains (Wright-Giemsa, Wright's, |
| Beakers (2) | Microscope slides | Quick-Dip) |
| Funnel (2) | | Whatman Filter Paper (2 sheets) |

## Inspection of Materials
### Microscope Slides

Slides must be pristine as a dirty slide will impede the smear making process. Inspect a slide by holding it up to the light, is it clear? Are there any spots on it? Discard any slides which are not completely clear. Store all clear slides in a slide box with the Student/Student Group name on it for use in Labs 5 and 6. Do not reuse slides or wash slides for reuse as artifacts will often be present.

## Staining Solution:

Staining solutions should be new, unexpired and devoid of precipitant. A quick inspection of the stock container of stains available will tell you if the stain is "tired" **(Figures 4-4A & B)**. Even stains that are within the expiration date can become tired or aged due to excessive use. To determine whether or not precipitate is present, identify two types of stain to be used in Labs 5 and 6 and procure both unused and used samples of each (i.e. Wright's, Wright-Giemsa, Stain # 1 of a Quik-Dip set) as a class experiment. Place a piece of Whatman filter paper within a funnel, suspend the funnel within a beaker. Set up two of these stations for each type of stain and label accordingly as Stain I-New, Stain I-Used, Stain II-New and Stain II-Used. Once the systems are set up, pour a small amount (5 to 10 mL) of each type of stain in the appropriate beaker and allow all of the stain to filter through the filter paper. Once completely strained through, with gloves on, lift the filter paper out and spread it out onto a non-absorbent, disposable paper to examine for precipitant. What do you see?

## Stain Station-Set-Up (secondary containers):

In preparation for Labs 5 and 6 secondary staining containers should be prepared. The ideal setup for blood smear staining is the use of Coplin Jars. These are manufactured both in glass or plastic with tightly sealed lids. Both are equally useful, however for such stains as Wright's or Wright-Giemsa, plastic will become discolored over time. The use of de-colorizer in small amounts is effective in cleaning glass jars and removing stain. Follow the instructions below to create staining stations for 2 methods of staining in Labs 5 and 6.

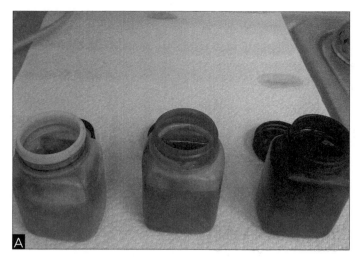
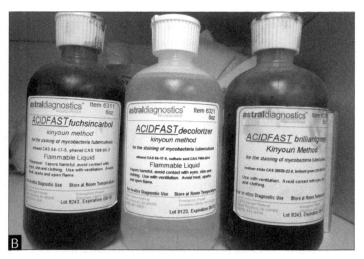

**Figure 4-4A & B:** Staining solutions should be properly labeled unlike this Dip-Quick set up pictured here. Stains should be labeled as to their content and the date when last changed (if used separately from the manufacturer's containers) or the expiration date. Old and dirty stains often leave precipitate or sometimes organisms that contaminate the stained slides invalidating the results (A). Properly labeled stain solutions complete with ingredients, manufacturer's labels and expiration dates can be seen with this acid- fast stain kit (B).

## Wright-Giemsa Staining Station:

i.  2 Coplin Jars
ii.  Water source for rinsing
iii.  Blotting paper (bibulous paper)
iv.  Absolute methyl alcohol
v.  Wright-Giemsa Stain
vi.  2 MSDS/SDS Labels (adhesive)
vii.  Sharpie® marker

1. Utilizing a stock solution label, create an MSDS/SDS label for each of the 2 chemicals used (stain and methyl alcohol) and attach it to a Coplin Jar. Also note the expiration date for the chemical on the jar.
2. Fill each Coplin Jar so that the chemical is just above the top of the slots.
3. Tighten the lids to prevent both spoilage and evaporation. HINT: Because methyl alcohol is volatile, expect a need to top off the container when it is opened in the next lab.

## Quik-Dip Stain (Diff-Quick): 3-part system:

i.  3 Coplin Jars or a 3-part vat (sold by Mercedes Medical)
ii.  Water source for rinsing
iii.  Blotting paper (bibulous paper)
iv.  3 MSDS/SDS Labels (adhesive)
v.  Sharpie® marker

1. Utilizing a stock solution label, create an MSDS/SDS label for each of the 3 chemicals used and attach them to the Coplin Jars or the 3-part vat. Also note the expiration date for the chemical on the jars.
2. Utilizing stock solution I, II and III, fill each jar with the appropriate solution to just above the slots.
3. Tighten all lids to prevent both spoilage and evaporation. HINT: The first solution (Solution # 1 – green) is alcohol based and highly volatile and will evaporate quickly if not sealed. Expect to have to top off the fluids often when opened in the next lab.

Ensure that both stations are near a water source as the last step of staining is to gently but thoroughly rinse the slides to remove excess stain. Set out blotting paper (bibulous paper) for gentle blotting of the slides. Also set out a supply of gloves and plastic disposable aprons for use while staining as these stains will permanently stain skin and clothing.

# LABORATORY 4 WORKSHEET

Answer the following questions to the best of your ability. Expect to utilize your laboratory manual, a textbook, and reference manuals.

1. Nucleated erythrocytes are found in:
   a. Ruminants and horses
   b. Dogs and cats
   c. Avian and reptiles
   d. Rodents

2. Nucleated erythrocytes when found in mammalian species may indicate which of the following:
   a. Anemia
   b. Release of immature erythrocytes (i.e. erythroblasts)
   c. Poisoning or toxicity
   d. A and B are both possible causes

3. Red blood cell rupture may occur as a result of:
   a. Forcing blood into the tube through a needle
   b. Struggling animal during venipuncture
   c. Needle gliding in and out of a vein during venipuncture
   d. All of the above

4. The "fight or flight" hormone that can be released when the animal is struggling is:
   a. Ephedrine
   b. Prostaglandin
   c. Estrogen
   d. Epinephrine

5. The breakdown of glycogen in the liver or muscle is known as:
   a. Glycolysis
   b. Glycogenesis
   c. Glycogenolysis
   d. None of the above

6. When using a butterfly catheter, what gauge needle(s) will do the least damage and aid in a smooth blood collection:
   a. 25, 26
   b. 20,22
   c. 18, 20
   d. 16, 22

7. Which is deemed a proper handling technique of a blood sample once drawn:
   a. Refrigerate for up to 24 hours
   b. Conduct all testing within two hours or less of collection
   c. Keep at room temperature on rocker for up to 12 hours
   d. Freeze whole blood samples if not able to complete testing within 4 hours

8. If a blood sample is refrigerated for over _____, artifacts may appear:
   a. 6 hours
   b. 8 hours
   c. 12 hours
   d. 16 hours

9. It is recommended when transferring stain from stock containers to secondary containers, that the _____ be placed on the secondary container.
   a. Manufacturer name
   b. Expiration date
   c. MSDS/SDS label
   d. A is not necessary, B and C are.

10. Precipitate matter may be seen on slides on which _____ is allowed to sit for an extended time before rinsing.
   a. Wright's Stain
   b. Diff-Quick
   c. Both of the above
   d. None of the above

11. When setting up the stains for this lab, the expiration date on the Wright's Stain is _____.
   a. EXPIRED
   b. NON-EXPIRED

12. The chemical used to fix slides before they are stained with Wright's Stain is called
_____.

13. The 3 solutions used for Diff-Quik (or Quik-Dip) are: _____, _____ and
_____.

14. Staining or filtering of Wright's Stain is done to remove _____.

# CHAPTER 5

## HEMATOLOGY – THE BLOOD SMEAR

# OBJECTIVES

This lab serves as an introduction to manual hematological methods beginning with the creation of a blood smear. The blood smear remains an integral part of the diagnostic protocol in the face of modern technology. Successful smear making depends on good lab practices beginning with the collection and ending with proper staining techniques.

This lab addresses the following Veterinary Technology Student Essential and Recommended Skills List as set forth by the AVMA-CVTEA in Appendix I, Section 6 – Laboratory Procedures Specimen Analysis to include:
✓ Prepare film and stain using a variety of techniques
✓ Prepare specimen for diagnostic purposes

# KEY TERMS

Aggregation
Anticoagulant
Crenation
EDTA
Eosinophils

Erythrocytes
Hemolysis
Leukocytes
Lymphocytes
Monocytes

Morphology
Neutrophils
Platelets Quik-Dip Stain
Romanowski-Type Stains
Wright-Giemsa Stain

# LAB 5

# INTRODUCTION

The blood smear when created properly allows the clinician a glimpse into the so called "River of Life" to examine the various cellular components of the circulatory system. It should be noted that proper collection and preservation methods in conjunction with the actual creation of a proper blood smear will provide a finished product to be used for staining and examination of individual blood cells.

## Discussion

According to the AVMA-CVTEA guidelines, entitled Veterinary Technology Student Essential and Recommended Skills List, Section 6: Laboratory Procedures – the veterinary technician should be fully capable of performing the following tasks when making a blood smear for hematological examination:
✓ Prepare the specimen for diagnostic purposes
✓ Prepare a blood film and stain using a variety of techniques
These directives include the following actions: safely restraining the animal to facilitate a smooth blood draw, drawing the blood sample aseptically and preserving blood appropriately. These actions all have the potential for determining the quality of the blood smear which is produced. For instance, improperly restrained animals may struggle which triggers hemolysis as a result of the needle slipping in and out of the vein with subsequent rupture of red blood cells and release of hemoglobin. There is also the possibility of injury to the person(s) restraining the animal and drawing the blood, and the animal if improperly handled. Alternately, hemolysis may occur if blood

is mishandled and forced into the tube; blood should never be forcefully "squirted" into collection tubes, but rather allowed to flow down the side of the uncapped tube.

Blood handling and preservation may also affect the usefulness of a preserved blood sample for making blood smears. The most commonly used preservative for blood is Ethylenediaminetetraacetic acid or EDTA; this may be found in the purple or lavender top tube **(Figure 5-1)**. This is not however, the only anticoagulant/preservative available. **Table 5-1** lists other commonly used solutions and corresponding tube/top colors **(Figure 5-2A-D)**. It is imperative that technicians be familiar with these tubes and what they may or may not be used for since this will affect test results. Although most anticoagulants will not affect the quality or results of a peripheral blood smear, other blood testing such as a complete blood count (CBC) or blood chemistry analysis may be affected by erroneous use of anticoagulants and bad choices. This is particularly true when dealing with mechanical analyzers (always check the manufacturers' instructions, using the wrong anticoagulants or chemicals, may damage the machine and void the warranty due to "misuse").

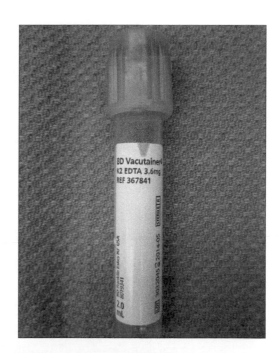

Figure 5-1: EDTA is one of the most common anticoagulants used when storing blood samples. EDTA tubes are commonly designated by the purple or lavender top as well as the label.

## TABLE 5-1
## Commonly Used Solutions And Tube/Top Colors

| TUBE COLOR | USE | ADDITIVES |
|---|---|---|
| Green | Chemistries | Heparin (sodium or lithium) |
| Purple (lavender) | Complete blood count | EDTA |
| Light blue | Platelets, coagulation | Citrate |
| Grey | Glucose | Potassium oxalate/sodium |
| Dark blue | Lead, trace minerals | Sodium heparin/EDTA |
| Red | Antibodies/drug testing | None |
| Light yellow | DNA/blood bank lead | Sodium polyanethol sulfonate/Acid Citrate Dextrose (ACD) |
| Red/Gray | Serum chemistries | Serum separator gel (no anticoagulant) |

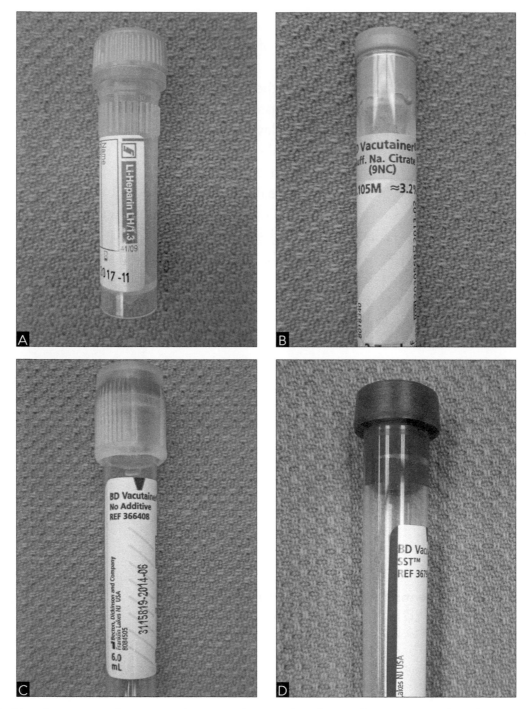

**Figure 5-2A-D:** Blood storage tubes come in many sizes and anticoagulant types and each serves a different purpose. Lithium heparin, or green top tube, is commonly used to store blood for chemistry evaluation (A). Citrate, or light blue top tube, is commonly used when evaluating platelets and coagulation parameters (B). No anticoagulant, red top tube, is also used for chemistries, antibody and some drug testing (C). Serum separator, red and grey top tube, is used to separate the blood cells from the serum for serum chemistry testing (D).

## The Order of the Draw:

Blood should be drawn from a calm patient in the following order: culture tubes, coagulation (light blue), non-additive tubes (red, red/gray) and lastly additive tubes (those with anticoagulants). The reason for this is to avoid needle driven contamination of chemicals transferred between tubes. If certain tubes are not required, simply remove these tubes from the order of the draw, leaving the remaining tubes in order.

## Labeling:

All tubes should be labeled with the animal's name, owner's last name, and date/time of draw, veterinarian's last name, and initials of the person drawing the sample. If the clinic assigns identification numbers to clients, this should also be included on the label. It is best to label tubes prior to drawing blood to avoid misidentification and always have extra tubes on hand in case of accidental breakage or loss of vacuum (in the case of vacutainers) **(Figure 5-3)**.

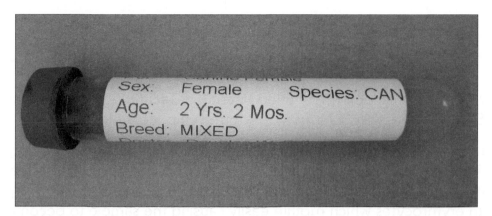

Sex: Female        Species: CAN
Age:  2 Yrs. 2 Mos.
Breed: MIXED

Figure 5-3: All blood or other bodily fluid and tissue samples should be labeled with the following: animal's name, owner's last name, and date/time of draw, veterinarian's last name, and initials of the person drawing the sample. Additional information may include the species, age and breed of animal as pictured here on this serum separator tube.

## Performing Venipuncture:

Students should review the methods and sites for drawing blood **(Figure 5-4)**, **(Table 5-2)**.

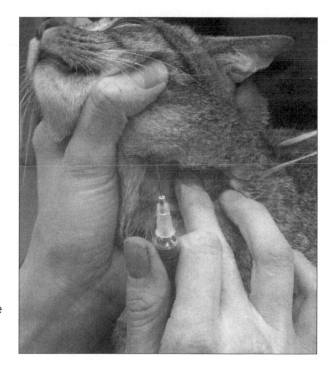

Figure 5-4: Blood may often be collected from multiple potential sites and depends on the animal and the phlebotomist's experience. One of the most common blood collection sites is from the jugular vein located on the ventral side of the neck. The phlebotomist is preparing to collect jugular vein blood on this cat.

| TABLE 5-2* Venipuncture Sites | |
|---|---|
| SPECIES | SITE OF VENIPUNCTURE |
| Dog | Cephalic, jugular, saphenous, sublingual, medial femoral |
| Cat | Cephalic, jugular, saphenous, medial femoral |
| Cow | Jugular, coccygeal |
| Horse | Jugular |
| Pig | Anterior vena cava, ear vein |
| Goat/Sheep | Jugular |

*As noted in AVMA-CVTEA guidelines, entitled Veterinary Technology Student Essential and Recommended Skills List, Section 3: Nursing (perform venipuncture).

Blood may be drawn using a needle and syringe or by the Vacutainer method. Regardless of the method used, it is essential to your success to use the correct gauge needle so that blood cells may be safely evacuated into the tube without risk of hemolysis (cell rupture). This is especially important when dealing with erythrocytes which rupture easily causing the sample to become hemolyzed.

## Making the Smear:
**Figure 5-5** demonstrates how to maneuver slides with your hands and instructions for making smears.

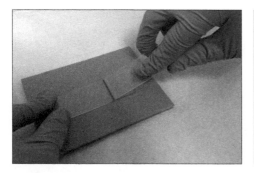 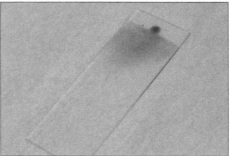 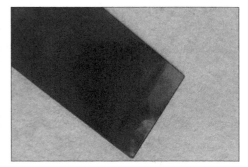

Figure 5-5: Procedure for making a proper blood smear.

1. Place a small drop of blood on one end of a clean slide.
2. Place the edge of the second slide in front of the drop of blood, back the second slide until it comes in contact with the blood droplet and stop.
3. Allow the blood to flow toward the right and left ends of the second slide until it almost reaches the end.
4. Push the first slide forward in one quick, smooth motion to form a thin film over the glass slide.
HINT: The size of the blood droplet directly influences smear thickness; start small!
HINT: Do not reuse the slider slide again, always begin with 2 new slides.

## Staining the Prepared Slide:
Once the blood smear is made, the slide should be allowed to air dry completely. The dried peripheral blood smear may be stained using a variety of stains. This lab will concentrate on two commonly used staining techniques. Quik-Dip (Mercedes Medical) and Wright-Giemsa Stain; **Box 1 and 2** provide instructions for use of both staining methods. Care should be taken not to contaminate the staining solutions while carrying out the staining process as well as wearing personal protective equipment (gloves, lab coat or apron) to prevent staining of hands and clothing.

# BOX 1
## Wright-Giemsa Staining Technique

## Introduction:

Wright-Giemsa stain is one of several stains which are generally used for examination of blood smears, cells and films. Careful preparation of the slide before and during the staining procedure is essential for the Romanowski-type stain to realize its full potential **(Figure 5-6A-E)**.

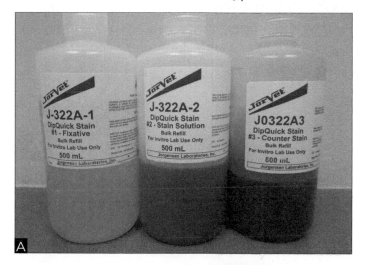

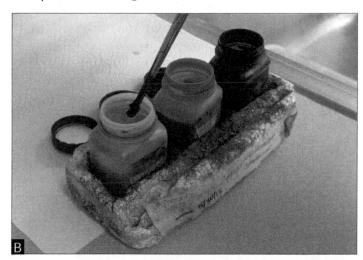

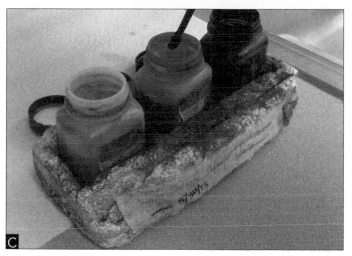

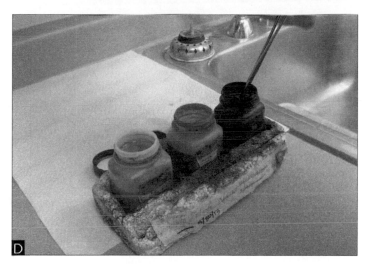

Figure 5-6A-E: The DipQuick stain set is commonly used for staining glass slides with fluids and tissues in veterinary practice (A). Depending on the manufacturer, the products may go by the following, and more, names: DipQuick (seen here), Diff-Quick and Quick-Dip™. This group of modified Wright-Giemsa stains is known as the Romanowski-type stains. All quick modified Wright-Giemsa stains generally follow the same slide staining pattern: 8 to 10 seconds in a fixative (B) followed by 8 to 10 seconds in a stain solution (C), then 8 to 10 seconds in a counterstain (D) and finally rinsing with water (E). The specific directions vary between the products and should be followed based on the manufacturer's recommendations.

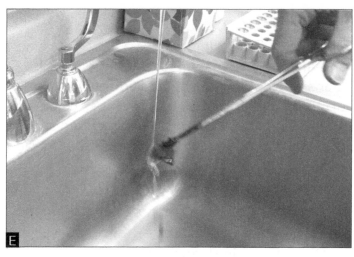

## Directions:
1. Fix the dry blood smear in absolute methyl alcohol for 3 to 5 minutes and allow it to completely dry, do not blot.
2. Place the fixed, dry slides in Wright-Giemsa Stain and leave for 30 minutes.
3. Remove the slide from the staining bottle, rinse it with water and dry (you may blot gently).
4. View the smear.

## Results:
You can expect to see the following cells stained well with Wright-Giemsa: leukocytes, erythrocytes and platelets. It is important to utilize the feathered end of the smear where you should encounter a mono-layer of cells without aggregation or clumping in evidence. Make particular note of irregular cells (i.e. crenation, multi-lobularization) **(Figure 5-7A&B)**.

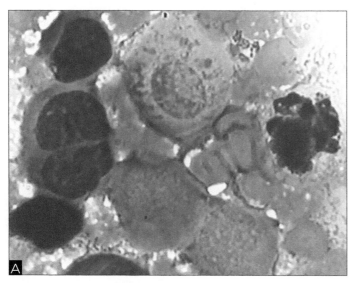 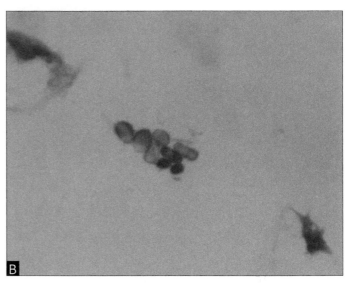

**Figure 5-7A-B:** Modified Wright-Giemsa stains are commonly used to stain blood components but can also be used to stain solid tissues, tumor cells (transitional cell carcinoma cancer cells [A]), spermatozoa, infectious organisms (yeast [B]) and more.

# BOX 2
## Quick-Dip Staining Set

## Introduction:
The Quick-Dip staining set is a 3-part staining set for the rapid differential staining of routine blood smears. It is also useful for microbiological staining of organisms and spermatozoa (*See* figure 5-7B). Consisting of a fixative, an acidophilic stain and a basophilic stain, Quik-Dip allows the staining for up to 50 slides in 30 seconds or less using a staining rack. Coplin jars may be used to stain 5 to 10 slides. It is important to clearly label secondary staining containers such as Coplin jars to avoid contamination. Results are comparable to Wright-Giemsa Stain methods.

## Directions:
1. Arrange the blood smears in a staining rack.
2. Dip 5 times in Reagent # 1 and drain on absorbent paper.
3. Dip 5 times in Reagent # 2 and drain on absorbent paper.

4. Dip 5 times in reagent # 3.

5. Rinse the slide rack under running water and allow the slides to air dry or use bibulous paper to carefully blot them dry.

## Results:
Since it is a 3-part system, variations in staining will occur. By varying the number of dips in steps 3 and 4, the intensity of reds and purples can be changed. Cells normally stain as follows:

✓ Platelets: Clear and visible;

✓ Eosinophils: Brilliant red;

✓ Neutrophils: Intensely purple nuclei/granules;

✓ Lymphocytes and Monocytes show colors within their characteristic morphology.

Stains become "tired" over time and will not stain as thoroughly. Always use fresh stains. Also, if the stain is contaminated because a slide was not dipped in the proper order, the stain should be discarded and replaced. Once the blood film is stained it may be viewed using the oil immersion objective of the microscope to identify erythrocytes, the different types of leukocytes, platelets and occasionally some protozoan parasites. Each of these cells and organisms has a distinct appearance and students should commit them to memory for ease of identification. Slides may be retained as part of the patient record or shipped out for confirmatory viewing as long as they are dry **(Figure 5-8)**.

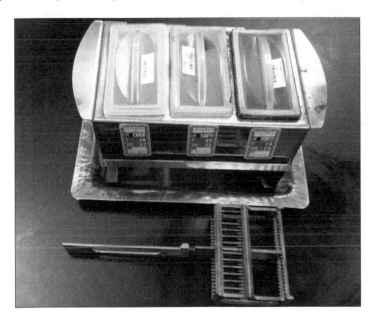

Figure 5-8: Quick-Dip secondary containers with slide dipping rack.

# LABORATORY SESSION

# LAB ASSIGNMENT
This laboratory session will allow students to become proficient in making a peripheral blood smear for staining and examination.

## Instructions:
Your instructor will demonstrate the proper procedure for making blood smears using blood collected from a mammal. Once you have observed the technique, refer to illustration 1 to compare

hand positioning of the slides. Using new slides, begin practicing your own technique. You should at the end of the hour have produced 6 slides of staining quality. What is a "staining quality" slide? The answer is simple: the blood should be smeared thinly enough so that cells are not clumped together or on top of one another when viewed, but rather distributed across the slide. The finished slide should be feathered at the ends, this is the area that you will examine when identifying cells. The photo below shows the feathered ends of a prepared slide **(Figure 5-9A & B)**.

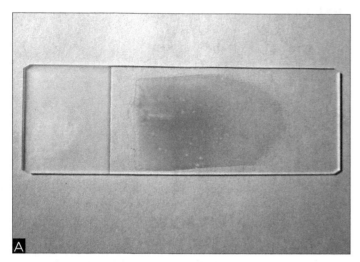 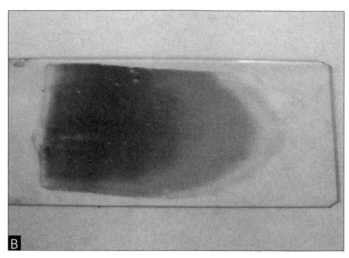

**Figure 5-9A-B:** Properly prepared blood 'stain quality' slides display an even film of blood tapering at one end with a feathered edge **(A)**. The same slide is then stained which better highlights the even distribution of blood and a feathered edge **(B)**.

1. Using the instructions found in Box 1 and 2, stain one slide utilizing each staining method. Store the remaining slides in your slide box for future labs involving white cell identification.
2. Observe the slide under the 10x objective, then the 40x objective and finally the oil immersion objective. The erythrocytes are the most numerous type of cell on the slide. Scan the slide and familiarize yourself with the erythrocyte comparing it to other cells.
3. Complete the worksheet titled Hematology – Smears, Stains and Erythrocytes.
4. Carefully wipe off oil and store slides in your slide box for future review by your instructor.

# WORKSHEET CHAPTER 5

## HEMATOLOGY-SMEARS, STAINS AND ERYTHROCYTES

1. Draw a representative sampling of the erythrocytes as seen using the following staining methods and viewed under the listed objectives, attach this page to the lab report as directed by your instructor.

| | | |
|---|---|---|
| 10x | 40x | Oil Immersion |

**QUIK-DIP**

| | | |
|---|---|---|
| 10x | 40x | Oil Immersion |

**WRIGHT-GIEMSA**

1. After utilizing both Quik-Dip and Wright-Giemsa staining methods, answer the following questions:
   a. Which method is quicker?
   b. Which method has more health hazards associated with the chemicals used?
   c. In your opinion, which staining method yields better results and why?

2. What are some of the advantages and disadvantages with each staining method?

3. How does "crenation" affect a blood smear, what exactly is this and what are some causes. Is it possible to prevent "crenation"?

# REFERENCES

1. Hendrix, C., & Sirois, M. (2007). Laboratory Procedures for Veterinary Technicians. St. Louis: Mosby-Elsevier.

2. NA. (2013, January 22). Retrieved from Clinical Pathology Samples for Hematology: https://www.vet.cornell.edu/animal-health-diagnostic-center/laboratories/clinical-pathology/samples-and-submissions/hematology

3. Russell-DeLucas, C. (2013, January 22). BrightHub. Retrieved from The Different Blood Tests & Tube Colors Used by Healthcare Professionals: https://www.pathlabs.org/clinicians/clinical-testing/clinical-tube-types/

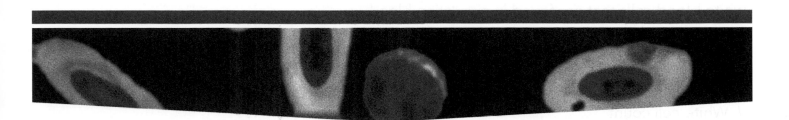

# CHAPTER 6

## HEMATOLOGY
## THE WHITE BLOOD CELL COUNT AND IDENTIFICATION

# OBJECTIVES

This lab is a continuation of the examination of the blood smear and an introduction to the differential leukocyte count as performed on a blood smear in order to identify the various types of white blood cells that are found in circulating blood.

This lab addresses the following Veterinary Technology Student Essential and Recommended Skills List as set forth by the AVMA-CVTEA in Appendix I, Section 6: laboratory Procedures Specimen Analysis to include:
√ White cell count
√ Perform leukocyte differential – normal vs. abnormal
√ Estimate platelet numbers
√ Calculate absolute values

# KEY TERMS

| | | |
|---|---|---|
| Agranulocyte | Hypochromasia | Nuclear hypersegmentation |
| Band Cells | Leukocyte | Nuclear hyposegmentation |
| Basophil | Lymphocyte | Polychromasia |
| Eosinophils | Monocyte | Thrombocytes |
| Granulocytes | Neutrophil | |

# LAB 6

# INTRODUCTION

Leukocytes are found in small numbers within the blood smear of a healthy animal; if seen in large numbers there is a possibility of infection within the body. There are a variety of leukocytes with each having a distinct and specific appearance. Students should pay particular attention to the size and shape of the nuclei in each type of leukocyte.

## Discussion

The word "leukocyte" is often considered synonymous with the phrase "white blood cells". There are several different types of leukocytes which are routinely seen on a peripheral blood smear; they are divided into two categories: granulocytes and agranulocytes. These cells are strikingly larger than erythrocytes (red blood cells) and normally occur in fewer numbers. While the average erythrocyte is 6 to 10 micrometers, the average leukocyte measures 8 to 20 micrometers depending on the type of white blood cell being measured. As a frame of reference, there are 24,500 micrometers in 1 inch or 10,000 micrometers in 1 centimeter!

The granulocytes are made up of basophils, eosinophils and neutrophils while the agranulocytes are made up of lymphocytes, monocytes and thrombocytes. An easy way to begin to remember the difference is the saying: "Men named Phil are grand sights" which reminds us that granulocytes all end in "phil". By process of elimination, any leukocytes whose name does not end in "phil" should be regarded as an agranulocyte. The major difference between these two types of leukocytes besides the word endings lies in the presence or absence of granules within the cytoplasm.

(Remember your medical terminology: a = no, none, without). The following is a short synopsis of the various types of leukocytes and some of their characteristics.

# Granulocytes
The subgroup of leukocytes whose cells contain visible granules within the cytoplasm. Each type of granulocyte name ends in "phil".

**Basophil:** A bi-lobular granulocyte that also has an irregularly shaped, pale nucleus. Granules seen within the cytoplasm of this granulocytic cell stain bluish-black and may be various sizes. This cell is normally seen in low numbers in the circulating blood (**Figure 6-1**).

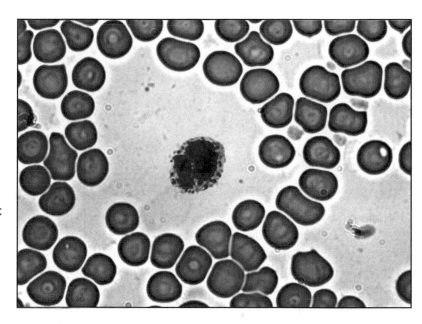

Figure 6-1: Basophils are relatively uncommon in normal blood smears and are character- ized by having two nuclear lobes, an irregular shaped pale nucleus and dark blue cytoplasmic granules. A canine basophil is shown here at 100x magnification. Note that the granules can be highly variable in basophils sometimes making them challenging to discern from other granulocytes.

**Eosinophil:** A bi-lobular granulocyte which traditionally exhibits a nucleus made up of two lobes connected with chromatin as well as rod-shaped granules within the cytoplasm. Eosinophil sizes and numbers vary according to species (**Figure 6-2**).

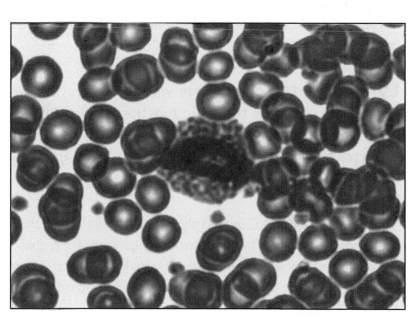

Figure 6-2: Eosinophils are normally seen in low numbers and are identified by a bilobed nucleus and pink to light purple rod to circular shaped cytoplasmic granules. A feline eosinophil is seen at 100x magnification. As with all blood cells, there can be significant variation of specific cellular details between different species depending on the health status of the animal.

**Neutrophil:** A type of granulated leukocyte with a multi-lobulated nucleus. The three to five lobes of the nucleus are connected by chromatin threads (made up of nucleic acid and proteins) and may also be referred to as a polymorphonuclear leukocyte. If the nucleus is undivided, displays no lobes and has no pathology, it is referred to as a band neutrophil. This is not to be confused with a hypo-segmented neutrophil which is seen in certain pathological cellular conditions (**Figure 6-3**).

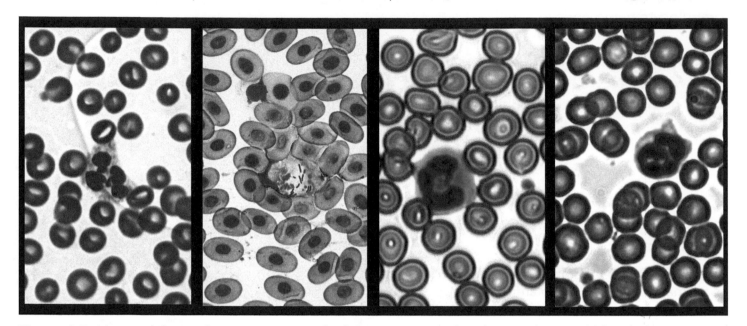

Figure 6-3: Neutrophils are the most common leukocytes in normal and most abnormal blood smears. Neutrophils vary significantly between species but generally have multiple nuclear lobes. Fish, reptiles and birds have heterophils (the non-mammalian equivalent of the neutrophil) that have prominent cytoplasmic granules. Mammals have fine cytoplasmic granules that may not be visible with standard microscopes. Infections and other illnesses can dramatically affect the appearance of neutrophils (and heterophils) as these cells rapidly respond to a number of diseases. To demonstrate the variations possible, several heterophils are shown: far left-capuchin monkey hyper-segmented neutrophil; middle left-sulcata tortoise with a toxic heterophil engulfing bacterial rods (sepsis); middle right-canine band neutrophil (immature and indicative of a 'left shift' response); far right-normal feline neutrophil. All images are 100x magnification.

# Agranulocytes

A type of leukocyte which does not display granules within the cytoplasm. The members of this group share the word ending of "cyte".

**Lymphocyte:** A leukocyte with a singular nucleus and no granules in the visible cytoplasm. Immune response is the main function of this cell (**Figure 6-4**).

**Monocyte:** A leukocyte that has a singular, kidney shaped nucleus. The major function of this cell is to act as a phagocyte (**Figure 6-5**).

**Thrombocyte:** Commonly called a "platelet", this agranulocyte is non-nucleated and disk-shaped in appearance. The function of this cell is clotting due to the ability of the cells to stick to uneven or damaged surfaces such as minor breaks in blood vessels. At any given time approximately 1/3 of the total platelets in the body are found in the spleen while the other 2/3 are circulating in the bloodstream (**Figure 6-6**).

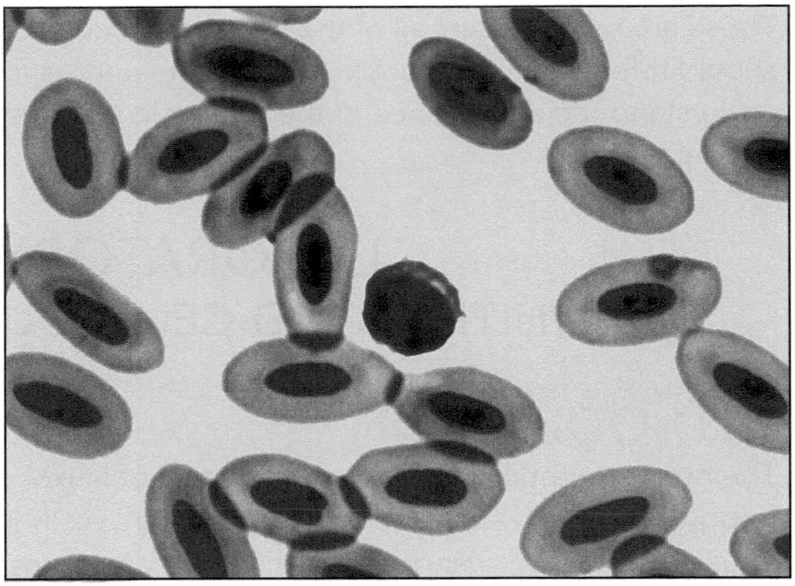

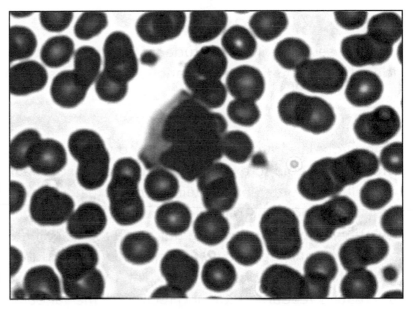

Figure 6-4: Lymphocytes are also common in normal, and some abnormal, blood smears and are characterized by a single round nucleus and relatively high nucleus to cytoplasm ratio. Golden eagle lymphocytes are typical of the same cell in most animals. That is relatively small, circular cells with a large round nucleus and smaller clear cytoplasm. 100x magnification.

Figure 6-5: Monocytes are occasionally seen in normal blood smears and are characterized by their large size (largest of the white blood cells), 'kidney bean' to variably shaped nucleus, and occasional vacuoles, other cells and even infectious organisms in their cytoloplasm. Monocytes work by phagocytizing dead tissue, cells and infectious organisms. A normal feline monocyte is seen here. Monocytes are generally much larger than lymphocytes, may or may not have clear vacuoles and ingested material and have a variably shaped nucleus. 100x magnification.

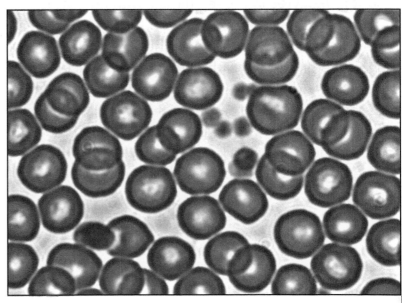

Figure 6-6: Thrombocytes are often the smallest cells found in normal blood smears. They may be found singly or in clumps but should be found scattered throughout a blood smear. Normal canine thrombocytes are smaller than red blood cells but can still vary a little in size. 100x magnification.

These are by no means all of the leukocyte varieties, but they are the most common. Students should refer to their textbook and other references for more detailed illustrations. It is important to understand the significance of the various leukocytes in order to comprehend the health status of the animal.

# LABORATORY SESSION
## THE WHITE BLOOD CELL COUNT AND IDENTIFICATION

# INTRODUCTION

The proper identification and enumeration of leukocytes is a valuable tool in diagnostic hematology. This is due to the various roles of these cells in maintaining a positive health status. It is equally important to understand the two major types of leukocytes and the cells that are associated with each. Students should endeavor to learn to recognize the various cells on sight.

# LAB ASSIGNMENT

This lab session will allow students the opportunity to examine stained slides in order to properly identify and enumerate the various leukocytes seen in peripheral blood.

# INSTRUCTIONS

Using your laboratory assignment and your textbook as well as other reference books (as provided), begin to examine a prepared blood smear that was previously stained using Quik-Dip as well as Wright-Giemsa stain (or prepare new slides, if needed). You should begin examining the smear under the microscope using 10x and advancing to 40x to count the leukocytes and identify the type. You will be utilizing a manual differential counter and performing what is known as a Differential Leukocyte Count or DLC. Although many of the mechanical hematology machines may automatically provide this count, manual counting is a strategic skill for a technician learning to create a readable slide and recognize the various types of leukocytes in order to provide hematological data for diagnostic purposes. Newer machine learning technology is also being used to count leukocytes in those animals with nucleated red blood cells such as birds, reptiles and fish.

Please take a moment to examine the manual counting device which (depending on the style) will have several buttons with corresponding pictures or text representing the various types of leukocytes. You will have to become used to pecking on the correct keys when counting cells. Do not despair, this is easily learned. Of interest, is the fact that most cell counters have a built in counter that sounds a bell when you have counted 100 leukocytes so that you can then record the various percentages of each type against the whole (**Figure 6-7**). These percentages will then represent the percentage of each type of cell in the circulating blood.

Complete the Worksheet for this laboratory assignment and submit it according to your instructor's wishes.

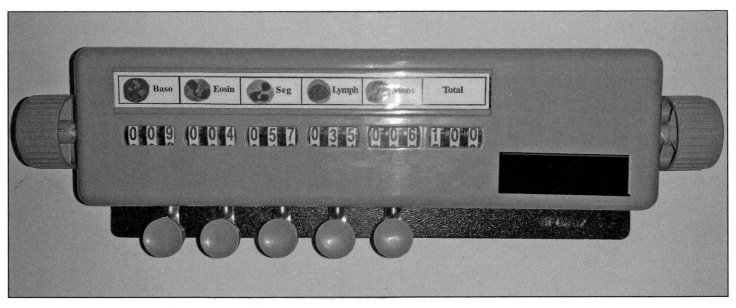

**Figure 6-7:** Manual cell counters are very beneficial when performing a white blood cell count. These counters typically make a noise, such as a bell ring, when 100 total cells have been counted.

# LABORATORY WORKSHEET
## WHITE BLOOD CELL COUNT AND IDENTIFICATION

1. Draw a representative sampling of the leukocytes as seen using the following staining methods and viewed under the listed microscope objectives, attach the page to the lab report as directed by your instructor. Try and identify the various types of leukocytes that you see based on nucleus shapes, presence of granules, etc.

10x

40x

# Quik-Dip

10x

40x

# Wright-Giemsa

1. After utilizing each of the staining techniques, which one is more convenient, which one generates the best diagnostic quality? Be specific in your answer._____

_____

_____

_____

_____

_____

_____

_____

2. After counting 100 leukocytes in each slide, fill out the chart below to indicate the percentage of the various cell types in the peripheral blood. Are the numbers within normal ranges? Discuss the results below. Use your text to ascertain the normal ranges for the species from which the blood comes.

| Type of Leukocyte | Quik-Dip Slide | Wright-Giemsa Slide |
|---|---|---|
| Granulocytes<br>-Basophil<br>-Eosinophil<br>-Neutrophil | | |

| | | |
|---|---|---|
| Agranulocytes<br>-Lymphocytes<br>-Monocytes<br>-Thrombocytes | | |

Discussion of Results: _____

_____

_____

_____

_____

_____

_____

_____

# REFERENCES

1. Hendrix, C., & Sirois, M. (2007). Laboratory Procedures for Veterinary Technicians. St. Louis: Mosby-Elsevier.
2. Studdart, V. G. (2012). Saunders comprehensive Veterinary Dictionary, 4th Edition. St. Louis: Elsevier-Saunders.
3. Thrall, M. W. (2012). Veterinary Hematology and Clinical Chemistry. Ames: Wiley-Blackwell.

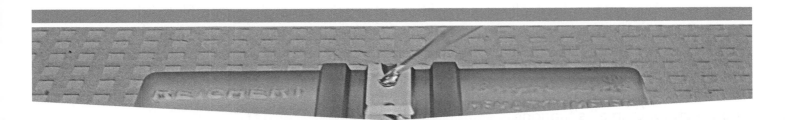

# CHAPTER 7

## THE 3 H's of HEMATOLOGY

# OBJECTIVES

This lab covers several manual hematological evaluations which are routinely performed as point of care (POC) testing in veterinary patients. Although the majority if not all of these tests may be performed mechanically as part of the automatic hematology "profile", it is important for students to be familiar with, if not proficient, performing these tests manually for two major reasons: a) the knowledge gained concerning how a test "works" allows students to understand the mechanics encountered when using hematology analyzers and b) developing a practiced diagnostic skill that may be useful when hematology analyzers are not available remains useful to the practitioner in all situations.

# KEY TERMS

Dilution Ratio
Eosinophil
Erythrocyte
Hemacytometer
Hematocrit
Heme

Hemoglobin
Hemolysis
Immune-Mediated Hemolytic
  Anemia
Leukocyte
Lysis

Packed Cell Volume
Platelet
Saponin
Unopette System

# LAB 7
# THE 3 H'S OF HEMATOLOGY

# INTRODUCTION

There are several manual tests that may be performed on blood as part of the hematological examination. Because every clinic may not have access to hematological analyzers, clinicians may expect technicians to be capable of performing manual hematological evaluations on patient specimens. Students began building a foundation for becoming proficient in manual hematological methods in Labs 3 and 4 as they learned to make a peripheral blood smear and stain it for the purpose of identifying erythrocytes as well as differentiating between the types of leukocytes found in circulating blood. Lab 5 allows the student to become proficient in performing the "3 H's" of hematology: Hematocrit, Hemoglobin and cell counts using the Hemacytometer.

## Discussion

According to the AVMA-CVTEA guidelines entitled Veterinary Technology Student Essential and Recommended Skills List, Section 6: Laboratory Procedures – the veterinary technician should be able to perform the following tests:

√ Hemoglobin determination
√ Packed cell volume (hematocrit)
√ RBC/WBC enumeration

In order to fulfill the educational challenge, this lab session will introduce the technician to the "3 H's" of Hematology and how the results of each test may be interpreted within veterinary medicine.

# Hemoglobin

Defined as: "a chemical compound within the red blood cell that has the ability to carry oxygen and carbon dioxide"; hemoglobin is made up of a substance called "heme" which in turn is comprised of iron (Fe) and globulins, a type of protein. As a medical determinant, it is important to measure hemoglobin in order to assess the concentration of oxygen within the tissue. This may be done either manually or mechanically. Manual examination of the hemoglobin levels may be completed using a hemoglobinometer. This hand-held device consists of the hemoglobinometer unit, an H-shaped clip and glass slide and cover slip.

In order to measure the hemoglobin concentration of a blood sample, it is necessary to force the erythrocyte to release the enclosed hemoglobin. This is done by using a saponin-coated applicator stick. Saponin is a plant-based material that has a sudsy quality similar to soap. It is derived from certain lilies as well as the soapwort plant and it naturally causes cell lysis. When blood is exposed to the saponin stick, the erythrocytes will experience hemolysis and release hemoglobin for measurement. The measurement is conducted through color matching.

The hemoglobinometer utilizes comparison of the sample to a standardized color panel built into the analyzer in order to estimate the hemoglobin concentration. It is also possible to establish the hemoglobin percentage in a sample using a hematology analyzer which operates on a photometric principle. Although the results are considered to be estimates, if equipment is properly maintained, results are deemed to be fairly accurate. Results are reported as g/dL (gram per deciliter of blood).

# Hematocrit

Defined as the "calibrated measurement of the percent of red blood cells present in blood" this test may be conducted manually or mechanically (using an automatic hematology analyzer); it is also referred to as the packed cell volume or "PCV". This test is especially useful in the assessment of the emergency patient and is often conducted in conjunction with total protein. An abnormal increase in the PCV may signify dehydration while an abnormal decrease in PCV may indicate anemia due to blood loss or internal bleeding, chronic immune-mediated hemolytic anemia, chronic disease or human error resulting from improper dilution factors or clots in the sample due to an improper anticoagulant ratio.

The hematocrit may be calculated using a plastic card reader, microhematocrit tubes and sealant clay **(Figure 7-1A-D)**. The sample must be collected and centrifuged before estimation of packed cell volume can take place. Results are reported as percentages (%) and represent the percent of erythrocytes in a circulating blood sample.

# Hemacytometer

The hemacytometer is a thickened glass slide with a thicker than normal cover glass **(Figure 7-2)**. The slide is permanently etched with a grid that is multifunctional for counting erythrocytes, leukocytes, eosinophils and platelets **(Figure 7-3)**. The hemacytometer is also used to count sperm when assessing for artificial insemination. Additionally, the hemacytometer is known as a Neubauer grid and it is necessary to utilize the Unopette System, or another dilution system, for lysing all cells except those which need to be counted. In this way the field is cleared of all cells except the ones of interest. It is important to recognize that each cell type requires a particular reagent-filled reservoir as well as a numbered pipette tip. **Table 7-1** lists the various reagents available from Unopette.

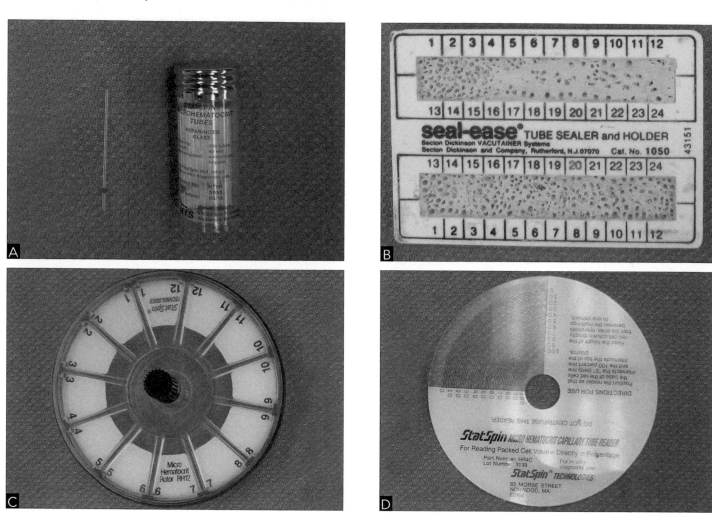

**Figure 7-1A-D:** The hematocrit (or packed cell volume 'PCV') is a measure of the amount of red blood cells in a given volume of blood. Blood is collected into a hematocrit tube (**A**) and then one end is sealed with clay (**B**). The tube is then placed into a centrifuge with the sealed end out in a protective holder (**C**). The spun tube is then measured on some type of card reader (**D**).

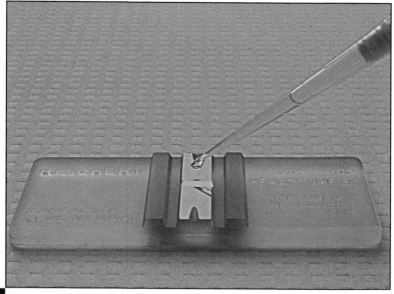

**Figure 7-2:** The hemacytometer is used for counting red blood cells, selected white blood cells and sperm. A pipette is being used to load the hemacytometer with prepared fluid (usually blood or semen). Modified from Wikipedia.com.

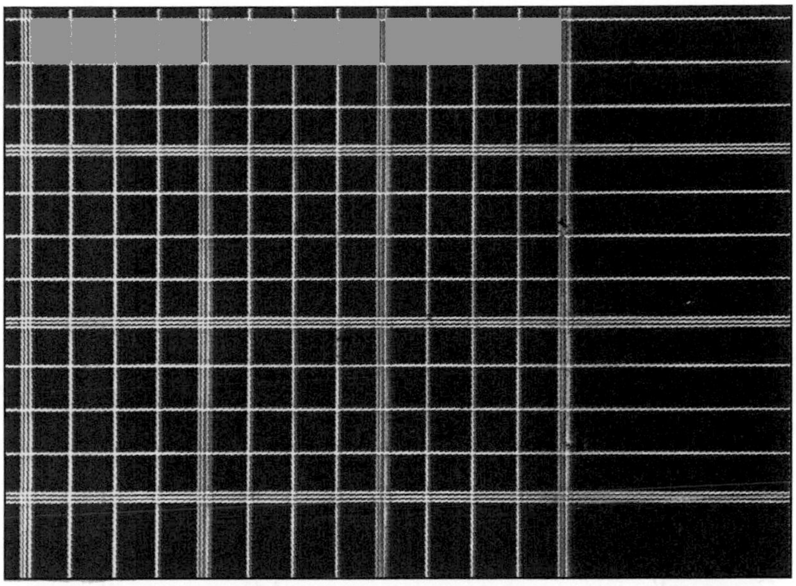

Figure 7-3: An empty hemacytometer grid as viewed under a microscope. When filled, cells appear and are counted using the grid system. By counting against the grid, cell counts are standardized and can be very accurate. When performed properly, cell counts using a hemacytometer are considered to be more accurate than those performed on a stained slide.

### TABLE 7-1
### The Unopette System

| CELL TYPE | REAGENT RESERVOIR | PIPETTE SIZE |
| --- | --- | --- |
| Erythrocyte (RBC) | Saline | 10 microliter |
| Leukocytes | Acetic acid | 20 microliter |
| Platelets | Acetic acid | 20 microliter |
| Eosinophil | Phloxine, propylene glycol | 25 microliter |

The pipette is designed to draw the appropriate amount of blood into the reservoir for mixing with the reagent to create the appropriate dilution ratio. Once the blood and reagent are mixed, the pipette is used to "load" the hemacytometer.

# Results

It is important to report results in an appropriate and universally recognized way. Hemoglobin is reported as g/dL, hematocrit or packed cell volume is reported in percentages (%) while the cells counted utilizing the hemacytometer are reported as a whole number using the following calculations:

## Erythrocytes:
Count the 5 fields; add the total and multiply by 10,000;

## Leukocytes:
Count the cells in 4 corners of the field and add them together, add 10% to that number and multiply by 100;

## Eosinophils:
Count 4 corners of the field and add them together, multiply by 2 then take that total and multiply by 8.8.

# CONCLUSION

The "3 H's" of hematology are useful as a monitoring tool for both wellness examinations and medical emergency situations. Because the normal ranges often vary, it behooves the student technician to commit these ranges to memory in order to quickly discern the abnormal and report it in a timely fashion.

# LAB 7
# THE "3 H'S" PERFORMED

## MATERIAL AND SUPPLIES LIST

Clip
Cover slip
Disposable pipettes
H-shaped moat slide
Hemacytometer

Hemoglobinometer
Micro-centrifuge
Micro-hematocrit slides
PCV card reader or plate reader

Saponin sticks
Sealant clay
Unopette or other dilution system for cell enumeration

## DISCUSSION

This lab will give students an introduction to the principals involved in conducting the following determinations: hemoglobin, hematocrit (PCV) and use of a hemocytometer for counting specific blood cells. Students will by the end of this lab be able to conduct each test correctly and report results appropriately. This lab assists students in becoming proficient in the AVMA-CVTEA mandated tasks related to hemoglobin, hematocrit and the use of the hemacytometer.

## Lab Assignment

Students will perform manual testing on blood to discover the current hemoglobin concentration, packed cell volume and number of erythrocytes, leukocytes, platelets and eosinophil's observed.

## Instructions
### Hemoglobin:

1. Lay a clean H-shaped slide flat on the table.
2. Using a pipette, place one drop of peripheral, preserved blood on one side of the chamber.
3. Holding a saponin stick, lightly roll it over the blood taking care not to displace the blood. Roll the stick until the blood resembles weak cherry Kool-Aid® then discard the stick.
4. Place a cover glass over the slide and gently ease the two pieces into the metal clip. Handle carefully to avoid dripping or spillage.
5. Place the clip into the side of the hemoglobinometer, seating it firmly.
6. Hold the hemoglobinometer towards a light source and look into the eye piece. You should see two sides of varying shades of green. One side is a stationary color standard (does not change) while the other side may be lightened and darkened by sliding the scale on the side of the apparatus. The object is to match the two sides as closely as possible. Once you are satisfied that you are as closely matched as possible, look at the slide rule and read the hemoglobin concentration at ____g/dL. The correct ruler for your reading is generally above the slide.

## Hematocrit (PCV):

1. Using peripheral, preserved blood, fill 2 micro-hematocrit tubes to the full mark at one end and seal the other end with sealant clay.
2. Place the micro-hematocrit tubes in a micro-hematocrit centrifuge unit with the plugged ends to the outer rim resting against the rubber gasket. Secure the lid to the machine according to the manufacturer's instructions. Remember to balance the centrifuge with an equal number of tubes or breakage will occur.
3. Centrifuge for 5 minutes.
4. Remove the tubes from the centrifuge and complete the PCV reading using Option 1 and Option 2.
5. Option 1: Using the hematocrit card follow the instructions as printed directly on the reader. Record readings on the Results page to be turned in to the instructor.
6. Option 2: Using the micro-hematocrit plate reader follow the instructions as printed directly on the reader. Record the readings on the Results page to be turned in to the instructor.

## Hemacytometer:

Due to the complexity of the preparation procedures for each of the cells to be counted using the Unopette system, refer to the next page for directions for proper preparation of samples and calculation instructions.

# HEMACYTOMETER SET-UP INSTRUCTIONS

## INTRODUCTION

The hemacytometer is actually made up of two parts, the counting chamber (resembling a thickened slide) and the thin cover slip which is specially designed for the purpose of use with the hemacytometer. Both should only be cleaned with deionized water; soap or other detergents should not be used as they may damage the slide or cover slip by leaving a film on the glass. The hemacytometer and cover slip should be stored in the case when not in use to prevent accidental damage.

## Instructions:

1. Ensure that the hemacytometer and the cover slip are clean and free of lint or other debris before use.
2. Prepare blood utilizing proper Unopette System or other diluent system for the purpose of "crenating" or rupturing all cells in the sample except those which you will be observing and counting. This is done by assembling the pipette system so that blood may be drawn into the Unopette container for mixing as well as destruction of all cells that are not to be counted. Do not use this for counting sperm.
3. Place the coverslip over the hemacytometer in preparation for receiving the sample.
4. Load the hemacytometer by placing the Unopette pipette tip at the groove on the slide and slowly let fluids flow under the coverslip. Caution: DO NOT OVERFILL.
5. Allow to stand for 5-10 minutes so that cells may settle.
6. View under the microscope using 10X and indentify the grid; this may take some focusing using both course and fine adjustment knobs.
7. Refer to diluent instructions regarding which parts of the grid you will count cells in.
8. The hemacytometer may also be used to count sperm that have been diluted with water.

# RESULTS

Date: _____

Animal ID: _____

Species: _____

Hemoglobin: _____

Hematocrit (PCV): _____

Erythrocyte count: _____

Leukocyte count: _____

Eosinophil count: _____

Platelet count: _____

# CASE DISCUSSION

_____

_____

_____

_____

_____

_____

# QUESTIONS

1. Compare the hematocrit reading using the card reader to the plate reader, are they different? If so, why do you think this is?

2. Create a chart listing normal values for the 3 H's for the following species: canine, feline, caprine, ovine, equine and bovine.

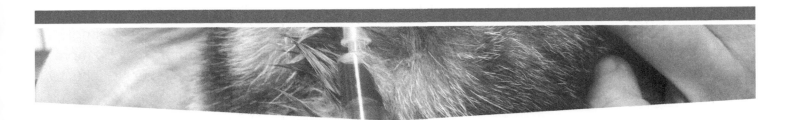

# CHAPTER 8

## COAGULATION TESTING

# OBJECTIVES

This lab introduces the student to the scientific principles and performance of coagulation testing in animal species. There are several factors which influence the proper coagulation of clotting as it occurs in the face of vascular clotting. Likewise, there are many different ways to ascertain whether or not clotting mechanisms are functioning properly. Some of the tests are fairly simple to complete and may even be considered point-of-care (POC) testing while others may be more complex in nature and require specialized machinery or supplies. This lab will expose students to testing methodologies which they may expect to encounter within a clinical setting.

This lab addresses the following Veterinary Technology Student Essential and Recommended Skills List as set forth by the AVMA-CVTEA in Appendix I, Section 6 – Specimen Analysis Tasks to include:

√ Coagulation Tests (one of the following must be performed)
  • Buccal Mucosal Bleeding Time (BMBT)
  • Activated Clotting Time (ACT)
  • Prothrombin time
  • Partial Thromboplastin Time (PTT)
  • Fibrinogen assay

# KEY TERMS

Activated Clotting Time
Autoimmune Thrombocytopenia
Clot
Clotting Factors
Coagulation
Coagulation Cascade
D-Dimer

Disseminated Intravascular Coagulation (DIC)
Extrinsic Pathway
Fibrin
Fibrinogen
Fibrinolysis
Hemostasis

Intrinsic Pathway
Partial Thromboplastin Time
Platelets
Prothrombin Time
Thrombin
Thrombosis
Von Willebrand's Disease

# INTRODUCTION

Students should spend time reviewing the science of coagulation so as to have a clear knowledge of the process and its importance. Only then can you fully appreciate the reasons behind performance of coagulation testing and the meaning of the results.

# DISCUSSION

It may be helpful to think of "coagulation" as a builder's process. When injury occurs, platelets are activated and travel to the site of the injury. They are responsible for releasing "factors" which in turn activate a "coagulation cascade". This cascade effect is one of enzyme activity and requires the presence of calcium and other components in order for the multiple reactions of coagulation to take place. These multiple reactions may be described as a "cascading effect"; hence one causes the next which causes the next, etc. The cascade effect is initiated through actions brought on by the released "factors" which are linked to the extrinsic and intrinsic pathways (Figure 8-1).

Once a platelet plug, or clot has formed, it must be stabilized. This is done by a product called "fibrin", a substance which holds the platelets together therefore supporting and stabilizing the clot.

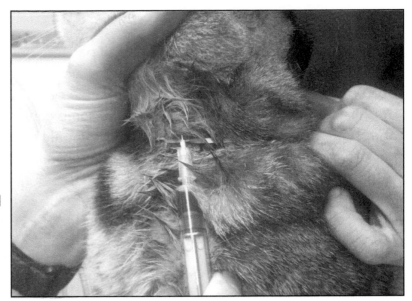

Figure 8-1: The coagulation cascade in a normal animal stops bleeding and allows for healing of a wound. This includes everything from minor wounds (as induced by collecting blood on this cat) to those caused by major skin trauma, surgery and more.

Fibrin is formed through the convergence of the factors of the extrinsic pathway as well as the intrinsic pathway and is not possible without the presence of the enzyme "thrombin" which is produced as a result of the coagulation cascade. Once the need for a clot has passed (due to a completed healing process) the process of fibrinolysis occurs (fibrin breakdown). This activity initially takes place at the edges of the clot to ensure that coagulation remains focused on the site of the injury. Fibrinolysis allows for clot dissolution so that normal blood flow can resume.

For quick reference, **Table 8-1** indicates the factors and cells that are assessed by the various coagulation testing methods.

## TABLE 8-1
### Coagulation Methods

| METHOD | FACTOR/CELL TYPE MEASURED |
|---|---|
| Platelet counting method | Platelet function |
| Activated Clotting Time (ACT) | Intrinsic and common pathway factors (all but factor VII) |
| Whole blood clotting time | Intrinsic clotting mechanism (factors XII, VI, IX and VIII) |
| Buccal mucosal bleeding time | Platelet function |
| Clot retraction | Intrinsic, extrinsic pathway factors XII, VI, IX, VIII, VII |
| Fibrinogen determination | Fibrin analysis |
| Prothrombin time test | Extrinsic pathway factor VII |
| Activated Partial Thromboplastin Time (PTT) d-dimer/Fibrin degradation products Factors VI, VII, IX, X | Protein induced by Vitamin K absence (PIVKA) Intrinsic pathway factor XII, VI, IX and VIII Clot degradation |

# CONCLUSION

Coagulation is inherently important to all patients but may be of special concern in cases involving physiological disorders, inherited diseases such a von Willebrand's Disease (involves Factor VIII), poisoning (certain rodenticides), autoimmune cell destruction (autoimmune thrombocytopenia) or physical trauma. Additionally, because some canine breeds (i.e. Doberman Pincher, German Shepherd, Golden Retriever, etc.) may commonly display inherited coagulation disorders, it is important for the veterinary technician to be familiar with and proficient in the common coagulation testing methods utilized clinically.

# LAB 8
# COAGULATION TESTING METHODS

## INTRODUCTION

This lab will allow students the chance to practice a variety of coagulation measurements as well as draw interpretative conclusions concerning the results. By the end of this lab, students will be proficient in the following coagulation testing methods:

√ Activated Clotting Time **(ACT)**
√ Whole blood clotting time
√ Buccal mucosal bleeding time
√ Clot retraction time
√ Fibrinogen determination test

## MATERIALS AND SUPPLIES

| | | |
|---|---|---|
| Blotting paper | Hot water bath | Sealant clay |
| Centrifuge | Incubator | Sharpie® marker |
| Diatomacious earth | Micro-hematocrit tubes | Syringe and needles |
| Disposable lancets | Refractometer | 10 x 75 mm tubes |
| Gauze for muzzle | Saline | Timer and clock |

## Lab Assignment

AVMA-CVTEA recommends that students participating in this activity work in groups, the class will be broken up into groups of 4 students. Two students will be responsible for restraint of the animal and drawing blood while the remaining two students will begin the immediate test procedures. Because of the need to utilize a hot water bath for three of the five tests to be covered, multiple tests may be conducted simultaneously. For this reason, all students should read through the lab completely and ensure that all supplies are available before beginning the testing.

Remember: The object of this lab is to test clotting ability. No anticoagulants are used; and timing is critical because the clotting cascade begins immediately upon drawing blood from the body.

All results should be recorded in the animal's records as well as on the results sheet. The results sheet and accompanying lab report will be submitted to the instructor for grading purposes.

## Activated Clotting Time (ACT):

1. INSTRUCTOR: Pre-lab Activity – Place 1 10 x 75 mm tube per group in a 37°C water bath approximately 30 minutes before starting the lab and allow the tubes to warm. The tubes should be labeled with a group name or number.
2. At the beginning of the lab – place a small amount of diatomaceous earth in the labeled tubes.
3. Draw 2 ml of blood in a syringe and immediately transfer it to the warmed tube, mixing gently before placing it back in the water bath, start the timer.
4. At 60 seconds, (after starting the timer) observe the tube for signs of clotting.
5. Continue to observe at 5 second intervals until clotting occurs (keeping up with total time). When clotting occurs, note the time and record.

## Whole Blood Clotting Time:

1. Rinse three labeled (1, 2, 3) 10 x 75 mm tubes with saline, discard the saline and set the tubes aside.
2. Draw 3 ml of blood and note the time that the blood appeared in the syringe.
3. Dispense 1 ml of blood into each of the pre-labeled tubes and place them in the 37°C degree water bath.
4. At 30 second intervals, tilt the first, second and then the third tube. Note when the clot forms in each of the three tubes.
5. Calculate the clotting time by noting the difference from the time that blood first appeared in the syringe to the time of clot formation in Tube #3.

## Buccal Mucosal Bleeding Time:

1. The animal should be allowed to rest comfortably while being gently restrained by one student.
2. A strip of gauze may be used to tie the upper lip back to reflect the mucous membranes **(Figure 8-2)**.
3. A 1 mm incision is made in the buccal mucosa with a lancet to allow free bleeding, note the time.
4. Using blotting (filter) paper, blot the first drop of blood away. Continue to blot at 5 second intervals until the mucosal surface no longer bleeds and record the time when bleeding stopped.
5. The results are measured as the amount of time it takes from puncture of the buccal mucosa until there is no active bleeding noted.

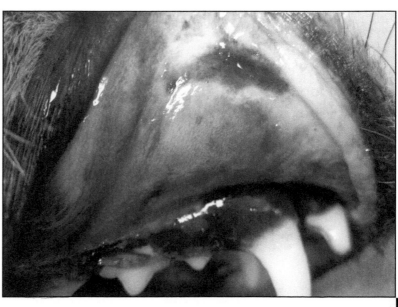

Figure 8-2: In preparation for a buccal mucosal bleeding time test, reflect the lips out of the way to expose the mucosa. The test measures platelet function. This dog has jaundice (yellow discoloration of the mucous membranes) due to advanced liver disease. Because low platelet counts are common with some forms of liver disease, the buccal mucosal bleeding time may be prolonged as was the case in this patient.

## Clot Retraction Test:

1. Draw 2 ml of blood and dispense into a labeled 10 x 75 mm tube and incubate in a 37°C water bath.
2. Re-examine in 60 minutes for clot retraction (clot will be visible and retracted away from the tube wall, almost free-floating).
3. Continue to examine at intervals over the course of the next 24 hours.
4. Note the time when the clot first appears, when it has retracted from the sides of the tube and when the clot is compact and almost free floating.

## Fibrinogen Determination:

1. Fill 2 micro-hematocrit tubes with blood, seal one end with sealant clay and centrifuge in the same manner as for a PCV reading.
2. Break open one tube to perform a Total Solids (TS) reading using the refractometer.
3. The second tube should be placed in an incubator at 58oC for three minutes.
4. Remove the second tube from incubator and re-centrifuge.
5. Measure the total solids following step # 2 above.
6. For each reading, multiply the TS reading by 1000 and report the concentration in mg/dL both for the non-incubated and the incubated tube.
7. To calculate Fibrinogen, use the following equation and the data obtained from step #6 above:
     TS mg/dl (non-incubated tube) – TS mg/dl (incubated tube) = Fibrinogen mg/dl.

# LAB 8 WORKSHEET

DATE: _____

Animal ID: _____

Species: _____

## 1. ACT:

Time (blood enters tube) _____

Time (blood clotted) _____

Time (reported) _____

## 2. Whole Blood Clotting Time:

Time (blood enters tube) _____

Time (blood clots Tube # 1) _____

Time (blood clots Tube # 2) _____

Time (blood clots Tube # 3) _____

Whole Blood Clotting Time _____

## 3. Buccal Mucosal Bleeding Time:

Time (blood first appears) _____

Time (no bleeding) _____

BMBT Reported Results _____

4. Clot Retraction Test:
Time blood drawn into tube      _____
Time (clot noticed)      _____
Time (clot retraction noted)      _____
Time (compact clot, floating noted)      _____

5. Fibrinogen Determination:
Total Solids (g/dL) x 1000 (non-incubated)      _____
Total Solids (g/dL) x 1000 (incubated)      _____
Fibrinogen Reading      _____

1. Complete a chart on the animal that compares all 5 clotting tests. Are the results markedly different? Why or why not?

2. Create a list (or chart) of normal values for each of the 5 tests for canines, felines and equines for quick reference.

3. Differentiate between the chemical and mechanical phases of blood coagulation. Be specific in your answer.

4. Create a chart that lists the designation, synonyms and what each factor (both extrinsic and intrinsic) affects in the body.

5. Explain von Willebrand's Disease, its mechanisms as well as identifying what breed(s) of dog is/are most susceptible.

# REFERENCES

1. Hendrix, C., & Sirois, M. (2007) Laboratory Procedures for Veterinary Technicians. St. Louis: Mosby-Elsevier.
2. Meyer, D. &. (2004). Evaluation of Hemostasis: Coagulation and Platelet Disorders. In D. &. Meyer, Veterinary Laboratory Medicine, 3rd Edition (pp. 117-119). St. Louis: Saunders.

# CHAPTER 9

## MECHANICAL HEMATOLOGY

# OBJECTIVES

This lab addresses the following Veterinary Technician Essential and Recommended Skills List as set forth by the AVMA-CVTEA in Appendix 1, Section 6: Laboratory Procedures.

√ Perform CBC (hemoglobin, packed cell volume, total protein, white cell count, red cell count)
√ Perform blood chemistry tests (BUN, glucose, common enzymes)

# KEY TERMS

Alanine Aminotransferase
Albumin
Alkaline Phosphatase
Amylase
Anticoagulant
Aspartate Aminotransferase
BUN (Blood Urea Nitrogen)
Calcium

Creatine Kinase
Creatinine
EDTA
Fibrinogen
Gamma Glutamyltransferase
Globulins
Glucose
Hemolysis

Heparin
Lipase
Magnesium
Plasma
Serum
Sodium
Total Protein
Uric Acid

# LAB 9
# MECHANICAL HEMATOLOGY

# INTRODUCTION

The use of machinery to perform hematological evaluations of blood specimens has become quite common within the veterinary clinic thereby negating the need to always send laboratory samples out to commercial labs. Bench top machines have in many cases replaced the use of such manual instruments as the hemacytometer, hemoglobinometer and refractometer which were covered in earlier labs. This does not mean that students should not be proficient in the use of manual methods; after all, what happens when there is no electricity, or the machinery goes down and must be repaired? Although the use of electronic hematological equipment is driven by spectrophotometric or photometric principles and will often generate more precise and accurate results, you should maintain your manual skills regarding hematological testing (especially in the area of the complete blood count) which may be useful when confirmatory testing is needed or out in the field with large animal patients.

Many commercially available machines are acceptable for routine in-house hematologic evaluations of common animal species. Commercial reference labs, however, may use larger, and significantly more expensive, machinery to handle the higher volume of samples that they typically handle. For the purpose of this lab, the use of the following equipment will be discussed:

- **IDEXX**
  - Lasercyte (complete blood count)
  - VetTest 8008 (blood chemistries)
  - VetStat (electrolytes and blood gases)

- **ABAXIS**
  - VS2 (blood chemistries, electrolytes, immunoassay and blood gases)

# DISCUSSION

Regardless of the type of machinery which is utilized in a clinic for ascertaining hematological values, there are certain principles that must be observed when collecting, handling and preserving blood samples. Beginning with the collection of the blood, animals should be kept calm and remain unexcited during the actual venipuncture attempt. When drawing blood, it is critical to avoid struggles as well as physical handling mishaps that may cause hemolysis of the sample. The sensitivity of the hematological machines is affected by hemolysis which will cause them to yield erroneous results or in some cases no results.

There are two methods routinely used for collection of blood: use of a syringe and needle or the use of Vacutainer® supplies; each is equally efficient. Though efficient, the blood collected by syringe must be gently placed into a test tube. To avoid hemolysis, remove the needle from the syringe before allowing the blood to flow gently down the side of the tube and mix with the anticoagulant **(Figure 9-1)**. Once the blood is in the tube, cap the tube and gently invert it to mix; **DO NOT SHAKE!** The use of the Vacutainer® method reduces handling and the possibility of hemolysis because the blood flows directly into the tube in a controlled manner as it enters the tube directly from the end of the needle **(Figure 9-2)**. The blood flow is controlled in such a way that only the appropriate amount of blood will enter the tube, this amount is in direct correlation to the amount of anticoagulant in the tube. It is important to mix the sample by gently inverting the tube to avoid rupturing red blood cells and causing hemolysis. **Table 9-1** lists tube colors as well as the anticoagulant that is enclosed and what tests may be run on the blood preserved with the various anticoagulants.

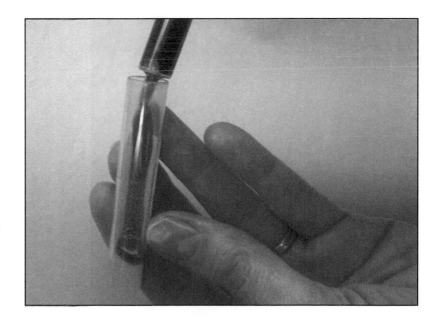

Figure 9-1: When transferring blood from the syringe to an appropriate collection tube, do not force blood through the needle into tube; rather remove the needle and allow blood to flow down the side of the tube. Blood that is forced through a needle will often have resulting hemolysis which should be avoided.

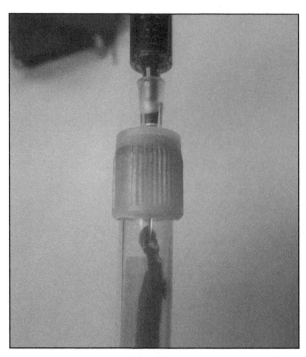

**Figure 9-2:** Vacutainer blood collection tubes have the air removed creating a vacuum. If using these tubes, the negative vacuum pressure will draw fluid into the tube using a needle alone. Again, it is best not to try to speed up the process by pressing the plunger and forcing blood through the needle which can rupture the cells.

## TABLE 9-1
## Tube Associative Colors And Anticoagulants

| CLASSIFICATION | ITEMS | ADDITIVE | TUBE COLOR | INTENDED USE |
| --- | --- | --- | --- | --- |
| Serum tube | No additive | None | Red | Clinical biochemistry, immunology and serology |
| Pro-coagulation tube | Clot activator | Coagulant | Red | Clinical biochemistry and immunology |
| Gel & Clot activator tube | Gel & Activator | Inert gel | Yellow | Clinical biochemistry and immunology |
| Plasma tube | Glucose tube | Potassium oxalate, sodium fluoride, EDTA/sodium fluoride | Gray | Glucose or lactate testing |
| PT tube | 0.109 mol/L sodium citrate 0.129 mol/L sodium Citrate | Sodium citrate | Blue | Coagulation testing |
| Heparin tube | Lithium heparin | Sodium heparin | Green | Clinical blood chemistries |
| Whole blood tube | EDTA tube | EDTA K2 | Purple | Whole blood hematology testing |
| ESR tube | EDTA K3 | Sodium citrate vacuum or dilute EDTA vacuum | Black | Red blood cell sedimentation rate test |

# LAB 9
# LAB SESSION: MECHANICAL HEMATOLOGY

## INTRODUCTION

To complete testing of blood utilizing both the IDEXX and the ABAXIS machines, students will assemble in groups of three. In order to allow students hands on training on both machines, consider utilizing the IDEXX system for the complete blood count **(Figure 9-3)**, and the ABAXIS system for the blood chemistries **(Figure 9-4)**. Students should consult manufacturer manuals for a list of supplies needed for each machine.

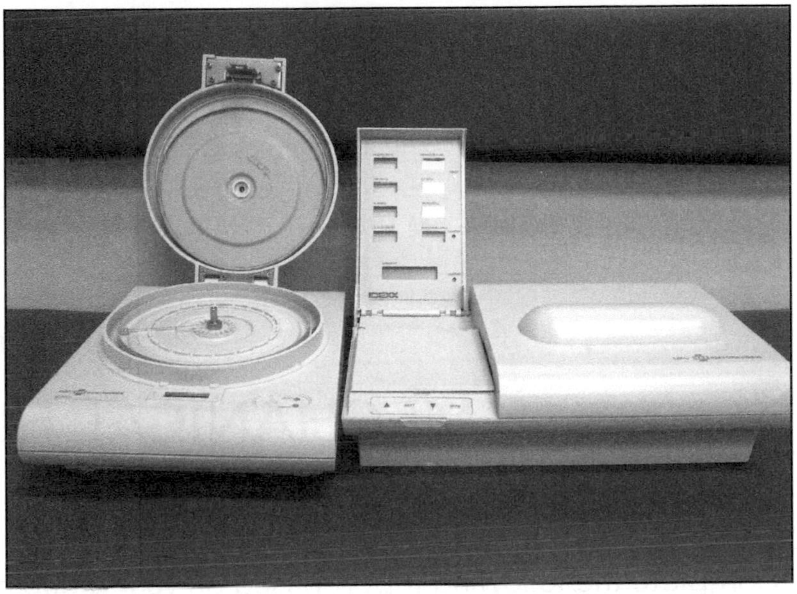

Figure 9-3: Automated machines such as this centrifuge and hematology unit can be used in small hospitals and provide fast reliable results for many common animal species. This particular unit can provide hematocrit, hemoglobin, white blood cell count, platelet count, fibrinogen and more results.

IDEXX: Lasercyte:
√ Blood sample collected in EDTA-K2 (*see* Table 9-1 for tube color)
√ Waste tube (yellow top)
 • The tubes for use in the Lasercyte are furnished by IDEXX and have a barcoded label, DO NOT use other tubes because the machine will not recognize them.

ABAXIS:
√ Blood sample collected in heparin (*see* Table 9-1 for tube color)
√ 1 test rotor
√ Pipetter and disposable pipette

The instructions for each machine are updated on a regular basis and your instructor will furnish copies of these instructions as well as orient you to the machines before you begin to run your blood samples. Pay close attention because each machine works in an entirely different manner and any deviation from the correct protocols will result in erroneous results.

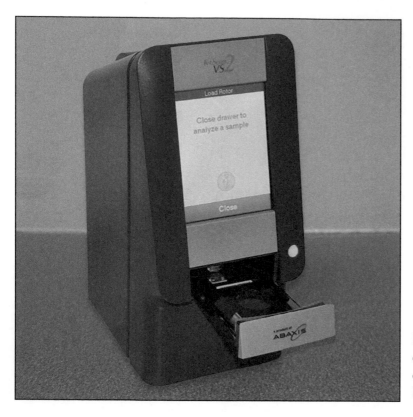

**Figure 9-4:** In house chemistry machines can often provide valuable results that can be obtained faster than if sent off to a commercial laboratory.

# LAB 9
# MECHANICAL HEMATOLOGY

## LAB REPORT

Complete the following report based on your groups sample results. Also, attach a copy of your results for both machines as provided by the machine's printer (IDEXX has an external printer connected to the system while ABAXIS has an internal printer which prints an adhesive strip).

Animal Species: _____

Animal Breed: _____

Animal ID: _____

Animal Sex: _____

Fasting Y/N: _____

Last Meal (date/time): _____

IDEXX CBC: Report all results (attach test results) and discuss possible reasons for any abnormalities (use more paper if needed). _____

_____

_____

_____

_____

ABAXIS VS2: Report all results (attach adhesive strip below) and discuss possible reasons for any abnormalities. _____

_____
_____
_____
_____

For overall testing, which hematology analyzer do you prefer, why? Also, briefly and in bullet format; note the pros and cons of each machine. _____

_____
_____
_____

Pros and Cons

IDEXX_____  _____

_____

ABAXIS_____

_____

# REFERENCES

1. Hendrix, C., & Sirois, M. (2007). Laboratory Procedures for Veterinary Technicians. St. Louis: Mosby-Elsevier.

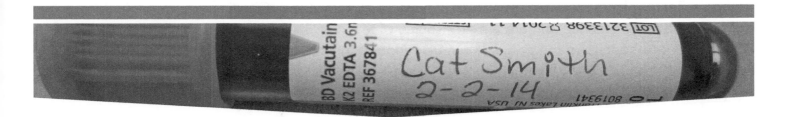

# CHAPTER 10

## ANTIGEN-ANTIBODY TESTING

## OBJECTIVES

This lab will introduce the student to the variety of antigen-antibody assay tests that are commercially available for detection of a variety of diseases and endoparasites which may be found in companion animals. Testing for such parasites as heartworms and the protozoa Giardia are commonly done within clinical veterinary practice and are a major source of revenue. They can also result in revenue loss if one does not understand the principles of utilization of the individual test kits and wastage occurs.

## KEY TERMS

Antibody

Antigen

Assay

Buffer

Conjugate

Control (Negative and Positive)

ELISA

Larvae

Microfilariae

Precipitate

Pre-Patent Period

Reagents

# LAB 10
# ANTIGEN-ANTIBODY TESTING

## INTRODUCTION

Antigen-antibody testing is commonly performed in veterinary clinical situations to identify the presence of a variety of parasites, viruses, bacteria, other disease-producing organisms and hormones. It is important that the veterinary technician be familiar with the technology that is involved in antigen-antibody testing so that they will be able to produce reliable results when conducting such tests on their patients.

## DISCUSSION

According to the AVMA-CVTEA guidelines entitled: Veterinary Technician Student Essential and Recommended Skills List, Section 6: Laboratory Procedures – the veterinary technician will perform ELISA, slide/card agglutinations, and identify blood parasites (*Dirofilaria sp./Dipetalonema sp.* – antigen kit) and perform diagnostic procedures for parasites utilizing the antigen kit.

The following test kits will be utilized during class (the instructor may substitute other kits which are already on hand):

√ Canine Heartworm Antigen Test Kit (Safepath Laboratories).

√ Giardia Antigen Detection Microwell ELISA Test Kit (Research, Inc.).

√ Canine Heartworm *Antigen-Anaplasma phagocytophilium, Borrelia burgdorferi-Ehrlichia canis* Antibody Test Kit (SNAP by IDEXX).

√ Canine Heartworm Antigen Test Kit (SNAP by IDEXX).

√ Feline Leukemia Virus Antigen Test Kit (SNAP by IDEXX).

√ Feline Leukemia Virus Antigen-Feline Immunodeficiency Virus Antibody Test Kit.

Each test kit utilizes whole blood which has been preserved using EDTA except for the Giardia Antigen Detection Microwell kit which requires fecal matter.

# Collection of Samples

Blood which is collected for this exercise must be preserved using EDTA. It should be maintained at room temperature for the testing and not refrigerated. If blood is refrigerated until it is tested, it must be allowed to reach room temperature before testing is attempted; placing the sample on a rocker will aid in consistent mixing of the specimen. A fresh sample is always best; however, test directions should be consulted for samples that are not immediately fresh **(Figure 10-1)**. Some testing may be conducted on samples that are 24 hours old as long as they are properly preserved and handled prior to testing.

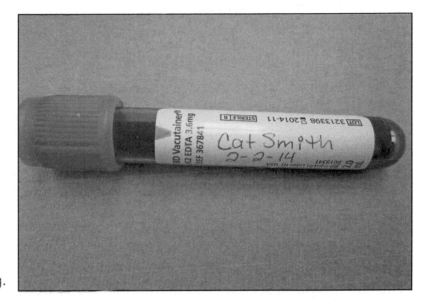

Figure 10-1: Before running any test, first read the directions to ensure that blood and other samples are stored in the appropriate container and at a proper temperature. This labeled EDTA tube contains blood for antigen-antibody testing.

Fecal matter should be collected as aseptically as possible. Because the test for Giardia requires such a small amount (pea sized) it is possible to either collect from the rectum or from a recently defecated sample. It is important not to utilize fecal matter that has been exposed to the elements because of the possibility of contamination by flies and other insects that may lay eggs in feces. These exogenous eggs may hatch and compromise the sample leading to erroneous results. Although it is understood that feces is not an aseptic biological product, care should be taken to preserve the integrity of the sample **(Figure 10-2)**. Fecal samples that are not to be utilized immediately should be refrigerated or may be frozen once (but only once) for later Giardia analysis.

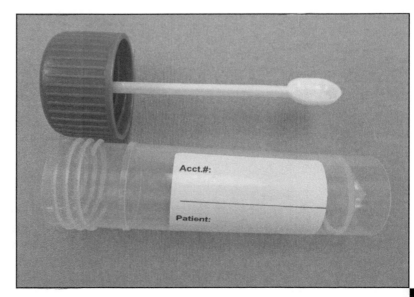

Figure 10-2: Numerous fecal sample containers are available. Samples can be stored in these containers, reducing the risk of contamination, for later testing if needed.

# Antigen-Antibody Testing

An antigen-antibody test kit will perform one of two functions; either it will detect antigens present on foreign or endogenous tissues or it will detect antibodies that are produced in response to an antigen **(Figures 10-3 and 10-4A-B)**. Let us consider the following protocol based on the need for antigen detection within a sample.

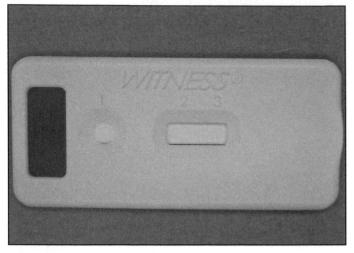

Figure 10-3: Here is an example of an antigen test that detects the presence of heartworm infection *(Dirofilaria immitis)*. The test kit provides a pipette that is used to draw anticoagulated whole blood, plasma or serum. A drop of blood is pipetted into well # 1.

The wall of the wells, tray or sample wand are coated with monoclonal antibodies. After adding a second enzyme labeled antibody, antigens in the sample come into contact with the coated container resulting in a color reaction. If there is no antigen present, there will be no color change. The same type of scenario occurs with antibody detection within a sample.

Many antigen-antibody tests are very sensitive and can detect minute quantities of antigen or antibody. As a result, sample contamination can easily result in false positive tests. This most commonly occurs when samples from multiple animals are being tested concurrently and cross contamination occurs. Student technicians should wash their hands or otherwise carefully clean them in between handling specimens from different animals, even if gloves are worn.

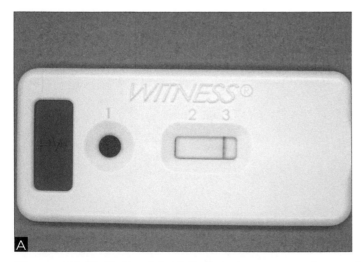
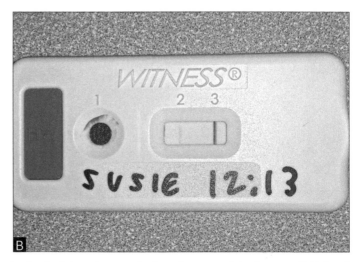

Figure 10-4A-B: Per labeled directions, an anticoagulated whole blood sample has been added to well # 1 of a heartworm antigen test. Sensitized particles bound to the heartworm antigens (if present within the blood sample) migrate along a nitrocellulose strip and the resulting complex forms a reaction along area #2. In example A, the single purple line along area #3 indicates a lack of the reaction and a negative test result. In example B, a faint line along # 2 plus the solid line along # 3 indicates a weak positive result.

# Conclusion

The success of antigen-antibody testing procedures begins with proper sample collection. This is followed by proper sample preservation and handling and ends with a technician who understands the technique and protocols necessary to carry out testing from beginning to end. It behooves the technician student to learn how to collect and perform antigen-antibody testing and the theory of antigen-antibody testing in order to assess results.

# LABORATORY SESSION – 10

## INTRODUCTION

Antigen-antibody testing is often performed within the clinical setting of a veterinary facility to diagnose the presence of parasites, viruses, bacteria, and other disease-producing organisms. It is only possible to ascertain correct results if testing is performed in an appropriate manner that is in keeping with the manufacturer's protocol. This requires familiarization with the manufacturer's directions in order to correctly run the test and interpret the results.

## MATERIAL AND SUPPLIES

Blood preserved with EDTA          Fecal matter          Antigen-Antibody kits with instructions

## Lab Assignment

This lab is designed to acquaint the student with the most common types of antigen-antibody testing, those which detect heartworms and feline leukemia. As an added bonus, manufacturers have packaged other testing methodologies with these two organisms so that one may test canines for heartworm, *Anaplasma phagocytophilium*, *Borrellia burgdorferi* and *Ehrlichia canis* as well as testing cats for feline leukemia and feline immunodeficiency virus. Not only does this act as a comprehensive health screening opportunity for companion animals, it is also a source of revenue for the clinic. Your instructor will supply the test kits that are available at your institution along with instructions for their use. This may vary from the kits listed previously in the lab and your instructor will advise you on this.

## Directions

The following test kits are to be utilized during this lab session and all directions are attached to this lab:

√ Canine Heartworm Antigen Test Kit (Safepath Laboratories).
√ Giardia Antigen Detection Microwell ELISA Test Kit (Research, Inc.).
√ Canine Heartworm *Antigen-Anaplasma phagocytophilium-Borrelia burgdorferi-Ehrlichia canis* Antibody Test Kit (SNAP by IDEXX).
√ Canine Heartworm Antigen Test Kit (SNAP by IDEXX).
√ Feline Leukemia Virus Antigen Test Kit (SNAP by IDEXX).
√ Feline Leukemia Virus Antigen-Feline Immunodeficiency Virus Antibody Test Kit.

It is important that students read all instructions associated with a test kit and lay out all supplies before beginning. Many of these tests are time sensitive and must be performed immediately from start to finish once initiated. It is also imperative that students ensure that they have the correct, properly preserved sample prior to testing.

Tests are invalidated in the following instances:
√ Wrong sample including cross-contamination.
√ Wrong or no blood preservative.
√ Expired test kit.
√ Wrong reagent.
√ Improper temperature of sample or reagents.
√ Mishandling of sample or test supplies.

## Results Reporting:
Test results are to be reported on the attached "Results" page.

# LABORATORY 10 RESULTS

Canine HW Antigen Test Kit (Safepath Laboratories) _____

Giardia Antigen Detection Microwell ELISA Test Kit (Research, Inc.) _____

Canine Heartworm *Antigen-Anaplasma phagocytophilium-Borrelia burgdorferi-Ehrlichia canis* Antibody Test Kit (SNAP by IDEXX) _____

Canine Heartworm Antigen Test Kit (SNAP by IDEXX) _____

Feline Leukemia Virus Antigen Test Kit (SNAP by IDEXX) _____

Feline Leukemia Virus Antigen-Feline Immunodeficiency Virus Antibody Test Kit _____

Questions: (Please attach, neatly typed, reference all external sources of information except test instructions): NOTE: Instructor may provide different questions based on kits/instruction availability. Students may also consult internet references to answer the questions below.

1. What substance is used by the Safepath Lab kit for heartworms to bind with the antigen and how does this substance contribute to the results?

2. In the Research Inc. Giardia test, what is the function of the horseradish peroxidase with thimerosal that is included within the kit? What part does it play in the testing methodology?

3. What is the purpose of the "chromogen" used in the Giardia test?

4. What is one possible reason for excessive coloration within the negative control in the Giardia test?

5. Discuss precipitation of solutions used within the Giardia test and how this may be handled.

6. Regarding the SNAP technology developed by IDEXX, what does color development in a patient sample spot indicate?

7. Regarding the SNAP technology developed by IDEXX what happens upon activation (i.e. snapping) of the device?

8. Regarding the SNAP test technology and the Canine Heartworm Antigen Test Kit, how would one interpret a test in which the negative control, positive control and patient sample spots display a color change? How would this be reported and what should be done next?

9. Discuss the significance of the low antigen levels and high antigen levels indicator spots on the Canine Heartworm Antigen Test Kit. How would this be explained to a client?

10. What is the most appropriate course of action if one observes background color that obscures the test spots? Why?

# CHAPTER 11

## COPROPHOLOGICAL TESTING OF GASTROINTESTINAL FUNCTION

# OBJECTIVES

This lab serves as an introduction to common laboratory procedures which may be conducted to assess the functional capabilities of the gastrointestinal system. Because the gastrointestinal system depends on many organs, such testing may be useful in assessing not only the common parts of the alimentary canal which extends from the mouth to the anus, but also the pancreas, gallbladder and to some extent the liver.

For species that have a cloaca, as with some exotic animals, fecal testing can provide insight into the status of the reproductive and urinary systems in addition to the gastrointestinal tract. A cloaca is a common collecting organ and end point for the gastrointestinal, reproductive and urinary tracts. As a result, matter from all three systems may be partially mixed together creating a 'dropping' that contains more than feces alone **(Figure 11-1)**. The individual components may be grossly distinguishable with normal samples but are greatly mixed with diarrhea and other abnormal conditions **(Figure 11-2)**. Birds, amphibians and some reptiles and mammals possess a cloaca.

This lab addresses the following Veterinary Technician Student Essential and Recommended Skills List as set forth by the AVMA-CVTEA in Appendix I, Section 6 – Laboratory Procedures to include:
√ Perform coprophologic testing

# KEY TERMS

| | | |
|---|---|---|
| Albumin | Folate | Liver |
| Alimentary Canal | Gallbladder | Mal-absorption |
| BUN | Gastrin | Mal-digestion |
| Cloaca | Lipase | Pancreas |
| Creatinine | Lipid | |

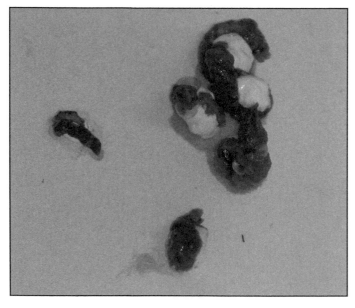

Figure 11-1: Normal dropping from a budgerigar *(Melopsittacus undulatus)*. The brown feces (digestive tract) and white urates (urinary tract) are readily visible. While common in droppings from other species, those that originate from arid land and/or eat dry foods may have little urine present. Sperm and other reproductive tract components may also be visible in normal droppings of some animals that possess a cloaca.

# INTRODUCTION

The gastrointestinal system has two major functions – to facilitate the absorption of nutrients from ingested food and to eliminate all waste products which remain after such absorption takes

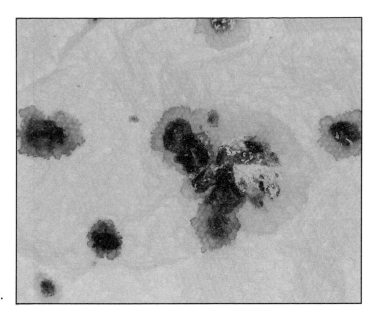

**Figure 11-2:** Droppings from a cockatiel *(Nymphicus hollandicus)* with hematuria (blood in the urine). It can be difficult to determine the source of the blood in the dropping as it is a collection of digestive, urinary and reproductive tract waste and/or secretions. The blood tinged urine and laboratory support of kidney disease helps identify the blood as coming from the urinary tract.

place. Specialized testing of both blood and fecal matter are essential when there is evidence of mal-digestion or mal-absorption taking place.

# DISCUSSION

According to the AVMA-CVTEA guidelines entitled Veterinary Technician Student Essential and Recommended Skills List, Section 6: Laboratory Procedures – the veterinary technician should be fully capable of performing the following tasks regarding coprophological testing:
√ Perform coprophological testing

Although the guidelines do not specify which test methodologies the student should be proficient in, it is important for the student to have a basic understanding of testing as it relates to mal-digestive and mal-absorptive disorders as well as parasitic syndromes that affect the gastrointestinal system. These tests would include (but are not be limited to) the following lab procedures for blood and fecal analysis as seen in **Table 11-1**.

Although this lab addresses coprophological testing of fecal material, it is equally important to consider hematological testing as a means of assessing functionality of such organs. The pancreas and liver both contribute to the homeostatic function of the gastrointestinal system, therefore the function of these organs should be assessed via hematological testing.

Fecal testing may be requested for situations ranging from gastrointestinal parasites to pancreatic insufficiency. It is important to note that although fecal collection is by no means a sanitary procedure, the collection and subsequent storage should be undertaken as aseptically as possible to avoid contamination. For this reason, collection should be performed so that exposure to the elements is minimized. Containers should have lids that render specimens air-tight to avoid drying **(Figure 11-3)**. Acceptable vessels for storage include zip-lock bags, plastic or glass containers. It is especially important (in litter or herd situations) that each sample be identified clearly with names, dates and case numbers (if appropriate) to avoid confusion by laboratory personnel receiving samples for testing. A specimen with no label or identification attached should be discarded as the results are deemed invalid.

## TABLE 11-1
## Testing Methodologies

| SPECIMEN | IN HOUSE TESTING | SPECIMENS OUTSOURCED TO EXTERNAL LABORATORIES |
|---|---|---|
| BLOOD | | |
| | Lipid absorption | Gastrin secretion |
| | Albumin | Fecal $\alpha$-protease inhibitor |
| | BUN | Blood folate levels |
| | Creatinine | Trypsin-like immunoreactivity |
| | Amylase | |
| | Lipase | |
| | Glucose | |
| | Bile acids | |
| | | |
| FECES | | |
| | Fecal floatation | Fecal acid-fast staining |
| | Fecal sedimentation | |
| | Acid-ether testing | |
| | Fecal neutral fat | |
| | Occult blood testing | |
| | Fecal cytology | |
| | Fecal direct testing | |

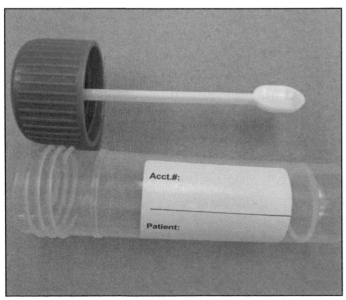

**Figure 11-3:** Fecal sample container. Several fecal sample containers are commercially available. All should provide an airtight compartment for holding the sample and a place to mark vital patient information for proper identification. In addition, this container is equipped with a spoon for more sanitary fecal collection.

# Collection of the Fecal Specimen
## Fecal Loops:
A fecal sample may be collected on dogs and cats utilizing a fecal loop or wand for parasite examination **(Figure 11-4)**. Before collection is attempted rectally, the wand should be lightly lubricated with K-Y Jelly which does not interfere with results. Loops should be cleansed and disinfected after use and may be stored in a mild solution of chlorhexidine to be rinsed prior to use.

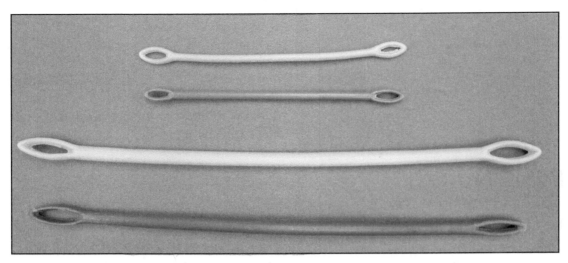

Figure 11-4: Fecal wands come in a variety of sizes and are commonly used in some clinics as a means to collect a fresh fecal sample. The wand is lightly lubricated with a water soluble lubricant and is inserted into the patient's rectum.

## Digital Fecal Extraction:
Often, upon expression of the anal glands, you may retrieve a small amount of fecal matter - do not contaminate the fecal sample with expressed anal gland material because it may affect fecal cytology results. Feces should be transferred immediately to a collection vessel for testing. Generally, the amount of feces collected in this manner from dogs will only yield enough fecal matter for tests such as a fecal float, occult blood test or fecal neutral fat determination, while larger animals such as cattle or horses will yield a significantly larger volume during rectal palpation.

## Environmental Collection:
Retrieving a fecal sample from the environment which the animal inhabits is not without risk of contamination. Depending on environmental factors such as insects, temperature and weather conditions, it is possible to unknowingly collect a contaminated specimen. Only when the animal a) produces samples (i.e., in a cage or kennel) immediately before collection or b) the animal is in an indoor facility with no chance of insect contamination (i.e., flies, beetles) should the sample be considered viable for testing.

# Fecal Sample Storage
Fecal samples should always be stored in an air-tight, sealed container **(Figure 11-5)**. If the sample is not to be examined immediately, it should be refrigerated until the testing is completed. This will slow or prevent egg hatch or larval development because of parasites and sample degradation.

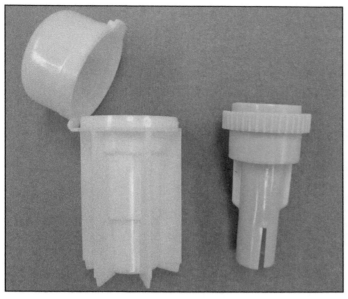

Figure 11-5: This disposable fecal sample container may be utilized both to collect the feces from the environment utilizing the green probe on the right and then storing in the white container. With this device, a fecal flotation test may be conducted by adding flotation solution to form a positive meniscus and top with a coverslip.

## CONCLUSION

Fecal collection and testing are two areas which are routine tasks for technicians working in clinical practice. The challenge is often in being able to collect a sample when you need it. Technicians should strive to perfect their collection techniques as well as their knowledge of preservation and testing methodologies. Good collection, preservation and testing methodologies are essential skills for the technician to develop and enhance. Understanding the implications of erroneous performance of these skills will allow technicians to shine as they complete these tasks to the best of their ability and therefore provide better care for the client.

# COPROPHOLOGICAL TESTING

## INTRODUCTION

Coprophological testing is often performed to rule out certain diseases, disorders and the presence of gastrointestinal parasites. It may also be done as a method of determining causes of mal-digestion and mal-absorption.

## MATERIAL AND SUPPLIES

Acetic acid
Applicator sticks
Centrifuge
Cheesecloth
Cover slips
Defibrinated blood
Ethanol

Ether
Fecal floatation solution
Filter paper
Glacial acetic acid
Gum guaiac solution
Hydrogen peroxide
Microscope

Microscope slides
Saline
Sudan dye
Tongue depressors
Water
Vials

## Lab Assignment

This lab is designed to acquaint students with the types of testing that may be done manually on fecal matter to determine not only gastrointestinal but overall health as it stems from the gastrointestinal tract and depending on the species, other systems. Below are the instructions for seven tests to be performed on fresh fecal matter. Fecal matter should be collected at the time testing is to take place if at all possible; refrigerate samples if not testing immediately.

## 1. Fecal Floatation: Detection of Parasite Ova:

Perform a fecal floatation in order to check for internal parasites. Place a small amount of fecal material in a vial and half fill the container with Fecasol®. Smash the mixture so that it forms a slurry before continuing to fill the container to the top with Fecasol® to form a positive meniscus. Place a microscope slide over the top of the container and leave it undisturbed for 10 minutes. Lift the microscope slide, turn it over with the fecal fluid on top and place a cover slip over the sample before placing it on the microscope stage to view. Begin at 4x, then progress to 10x to scan slide for ova. Identify any parasitic ova that you see and draw them in the circle on the results page **(Figures 11-6 through 11-8)**.

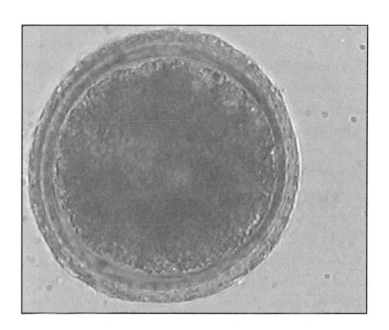

**Figure 11-6:** Canine roundworm egg seen on standard fecal floatation. Roundworms are considered zoonotic. All tissue, and especially fecal, samples should be handled with care to prevent contamination of the sample and exposure to potentially infectious agents. Clients of animals with known zoonotic diseases should also be counseled about risks and proper treatment.

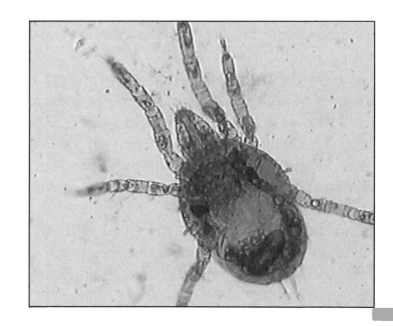

**Figure 11-7:** A non-parasitic mite found in the stool of a cat on fecal floatation. This mite may have been present on one of the food items the cat was eating. Sometimes skin parasites can be found in the stool when animals intentionally or accidentally consume them during grooming.

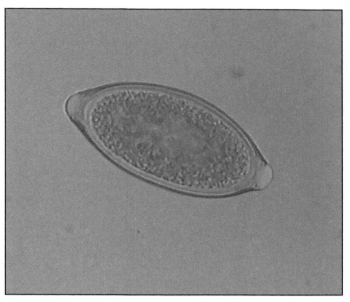

**Figure 11-8:** Whipworm egg found in a dog's stool on fecal floatation. Some parasites intermittently shed ova and can give false negative results. Whipworm ova of many species are shed intermittently and may be found adhered to perianal tissue and not just in the stool.

## 2. Sedimentation Test: Detection of Parasite Ova:

Mix 1 gram of feces with 40 mL of water or saline in a beaker making certain that the feces are totally crushed in order to free any ova present before pouring the mixture into a centrifuge tube. Centrifuge for 4 minutes before pouring off the supernatant fluid. Collect a small amount of the sediment with a pipette and place it on a microscope slide, apply a cover slip and view beginning at 4x, then moving to 10x and if necessary 40x. Note and draw any organisms/ova that you see on the results page.

## 3. Acid-Ether Test: Sedimentation Examination:

In a test tube, combine 10 mL of acetic acid with 1 gram of feces and mix, thoroughly crushing feces. Strain the mixture through cheesecloth into a centrifuge tube. Add 10 ml of ether to the mixture, cover and shake the tube to mix thoroughly; then centrifuge for 2 minutes. When removed from centrifuge, the tube should have 4 distinct layers: ether (top layer), fecal plug, acid solution and sediment (bottom). Discard the first three layers carefully with the use of an applicator stick before removing a small amount of the sediment and placing it onto a microscope slide. Place a cover slip over the sample for viewing under the microscope. Begin at the lowest power and focus while scanning for parasite ova before moving on to the 10x as well as 40x if needed. Note your findings and draw any organisms that you may see on the results page.

## 4. Fecal Neutral Fat: Presence of Fat in Feces:

Place a sample of fresh fecal matter on a microscope slide and add 2 drops of water before mixing well with an applicator stick. Add 2 drops of Ethanol and several drops of Sudan Dye (3 to 4 drops) and mix well. Place a cover slip over the sample and examine under microscope at 4 or 10x for red-orange droplets. What are these droplets and what is their significance when found in a fecal sample? Record your answers on the results page.

## 5. Occult Blood Test: Fecal Blood:

Smear fecal matter sparingly on 1 piece of filter paper. Label a separate piece of filter paper as the control by placing one drop of fresh or defibrinated blood (blood that has been preserved with an anticoagulant) onto the middle of the filter paper. To each piece of paper, add 2 drops each of glacial acetic acid, gum guaiac solution and hydrogen peroxide to each sample. Observe for a color change as noted below and record the results on your results page as well as the possible reasons for the color changes based on the animal's health history.

| READING | COLOR CHANGE |
|---|---|
| Trace | Faint green-blue appearance in approx. 1 minute |
| 1+ | Light blue appearance slow in appearing |
| 2+ | Clear blue appearing fairly fast |
| 3+ | Deep blue appearing almost immediately |
| 4+ | Deep blue immediately, no delay |
| CONTROL | Should display a reading of 1+ |

## 6. Fecal Direct Test: Detection of Ova and Motile Parasites:

Smear a small amount of fresh feces on a plain glass slide (**Figure 11-9**). Put 1 to 2 drops of 0.9% saline (standard NaCl solution) on the smeared feces and mix well creating a thin solution. Place a coverslip over the feces saline mixture. Scan the cover slipped area under 10x for ova and motile organisms. Increase the objective to 40x to more closely scan for motile organisms and small ova. Note as well as draw any organisms that you may see on the results page.

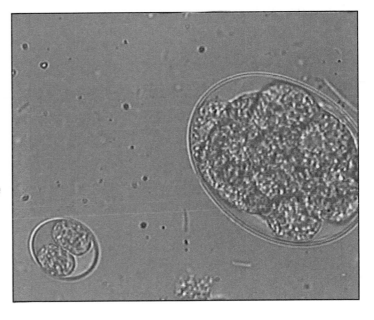

Figure 11-9: In addition to motile bacteria and protozoa (best demonstrated via video), some parasitic ova can be found on direct fecal examination. Here coccidia (lower left) and hookworm oocysts (upper right) were found in a finch's stool sample on direct examination. A small amount of fresh feces or dropping is placed on a slide, gently mixed with saline, covered with a coverslip and viewed under the microscope.

## 7. Fecal Cytology: Detection of Blood, Inflammation and Characterization of Fecal Inhabitants:

Using a small wooden dowel (i.e., wood end of a cotton tip applicator), smear a thin layer of feces on a plain glass slide (**Figure 11-10**). It is important to note that clumps or thick layers will result in uneven staining. Allow the slide to air dry. Stain the slide per directions of the stain system. Common stains include Wright-Giemsa, Gram and acid-fast. Each stain is designed to highlight different aspects of the stained cells, organisms or non-organic components and therefore serve different functions. Record your observations on the results page keeping in mind the function of the stain used.

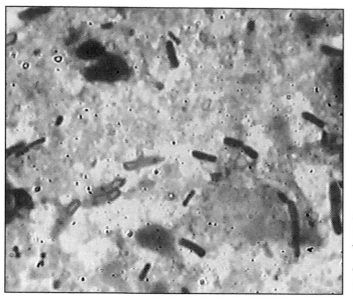

**Figure 11-10:** Fecal cytology of a ferret with diarrhea. Numerous large rods with spores on the end are seen. While not diagnostic, this is supportive of a clostridial diarrhea (caused by the Clostridium sp. family of bacteria).

# RESULTS

FECAL FLOATATION:

_____
_____
_____

SEDIMENTATION TEST:

_____
_____
_____
_____

ACID-ETHER TEST:

_____
_____
_____
_____

FECAL NEUTRAL FAT:

_____
_____
_____
_____

OCCULT BLOOD TEST:

_____
_____
_____

**FECAL DIRECT TEST:**

_____

_____

_____

_____

**FECAL CYTOLOGY:**

_____

_____

_____

_____

# REFERENCES

1. Hendrix, C., & Robinson, E. (2012). Diagnostic Parasitology for Veterinary Technicians. St. Louis: Elsevier-Mosby.
2. Rosenfeld, A. (2010). Clinical Pathology for the Veterinary Team. Ames: Wiley-Blackwell.

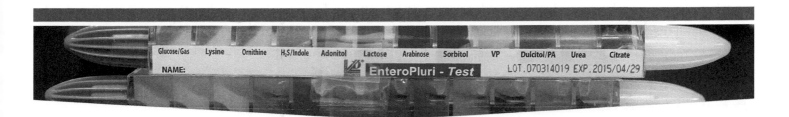

# CHAPTER 12

## MICROBIOLOGICAL PREPARATION

# OBJECTIVES

This lab introduces the student to the in-house microbiological lab bench as well as the variety of media available to work with. In order to perform microbiological veterinary tasks in a clinical setting, you must have a dedicated lab area which allows for specimen collection, processing and analysis. This lab serves as a microbiological "preamble" in terms of AVMA –CVTEA requirements while Chapters 13 and 14 will address specific recommended skills.

# KEY TERMS

Agar
Analytical Balance
Asepsis
Broth
Carbon
Contaminants
Contamination
Defibrinated
Dehydrated Media

Differential Media
Energy
Enteric Pathogen
Enterotube II®
Fastidious Organism
Fungassay®
Gelatin
Growth Factors
Media

Microbes
Micro-Organisms
Minerals
Nitrogen
Selective Media
Slants
Staphylococcus
Vitamins

# INTRODUCTION

The use of microbiological techniques in the clinical veterinary practice is often understated and overlooked by practitioners. This is partly due to a lack of personnel who while trained, may lack initiative or interest in maintaining a dedicated, in-house microbiology bench or due to the expense of such an endeavor combined with the ease of utilizing an outside laboratory to receive "send-out" microbiological samples. If there is an interest and willingness to undertake such a project, veterinary microbiology can be a rewarding, challenging and financially lucrative endeavor for any practice, large or small.

# DISCUSSION

While the study of microbiology is in itself a rigorous discipline, it may be reduced in its complexity for the veterinary technician student to a level of understanding that allows for the development of clinical aptitude (as required by AVMA-CVTEA guidelines). Those who become engaged and have an interest in this area of clinical laboratory science as it pertains to veterinary medicine may find a myriad of career choices ranging from clinical practice to regulatory or laboratory settings for their consideration.

The clinical setting does not generally have a large amount of space for laboratory needs since most space is dedicated to clinical care and treatment. Because of the minimal equipment needed for clinical microbiology, one can perform many types of analyses in a small dedicated space.

## The Clinical Microbiology Bench

The most important aspect of a dedicated microbiology bench is the need to maintain aseptic cleanliness at all times. By the very nature of microbiology, one must have a bench of pristine cleanliness in which to plate and examine specimens suspected of microbial contamination. To attempt microbiological work in anything less, invites misidentification of the microbes present and therefore the possibility of misdiagnosis and treatment. The same is true of the preparation of growth media; chiefly agars and broths used for sample inoculation.

# Media Preparation and Usage

The use of media is essential in microbiological applications in which the media chosen must be conducive to the environmental well-being of the suspect bacteria or other microbe. With this in mind, it is important to recognize seven key nutritional requirements for most microbial survival: carbon, energy, nitrogen, minerals, vitamins, growth factors and water. These components are readily supplied in media agars and broths which may be selective media (allows some bacteria to grow while inhibiting others) or differential media (contains substances which allow distinct and different bacterial appearances). For this reason, you must have a basic understanding of which media can be used and when. There are many different types of media available at a variety of prices and packaging **(Figure 12-1)**.

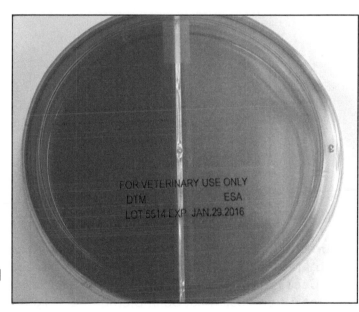

Figure 12-1: Dehydrated, liquid and solid media are available for many different types of microbiologic assays. Shown here are two solid media (Dermatophyte Test Medium and Enhanced Sporulation Agar) packaged together and used for dermatophyte growth.

# Media Types
## Dehydrated Media:

Sold in powder or granular form, dehydrated media has the advantages of long shelf life, ease of storage and the ability to be purchased in large quantity containers. The disadvantage of both dehydrated agar as well as broth is that for solid agar plates, you must have access to precise measurement scales such as an analytical balance in order to guarantee a mixture which ultimately becomes a solid gel (when properly prepared). Sterilization is also a major factor in the preparation of this product and aseptic sterile technique must be practiced, to ensure a usable product.

## Liquid Media:

Sold in sealed bottles, this media is used for broth applications and is convenient to use because it is pre-mixed and ready-to-pour. With good aseptic technique, broth media are excellent for tube cultures.

## Solid (gel) Media:

Sold in sealed bottles, solid media must be heated to its melting point using a hot water bath or other device (i.e. microwave), so that it can be poured into either petri dishes or slant tubes. Aseptic control is not difficult however there is a safety factor to consider because it is possible to sustain burns in the heating and pouring of this media due to the high temperature that is needed to completely liquefy the media.

## Commercially Prepared Agar Plates and Tubes:

Commercially prepared microbiology agars have replaced (to a large degree) the need for dehydrated media in many labs, especially where few microbiological studies are conducted **(Figure 12-2)**. A quick search on the Internet reveals an abundance of companies offering ready-made, sterile media in petri dishes and tubes in a wide assortment of types, both differential and selective. The option of utilizing such media is attractive for clinical applications because they are inexpensive and easy to store and use. If not used often they do dry out over an extended period of time, especially if retained past the expiration date; dried or expired products should be discarded.

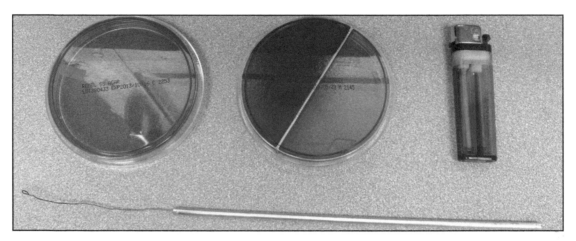

Figure 12-2: Salmonella/Shigella *(left)* and Blood and MacConkey's agar plates *(right)* are commonly used in clinical practice. These types of commercially prepared plates are readily available, affordable and easy to use. Because the agar is already prepared and can rapidly degrade if handled improperly, certain precautions on storage and use must be implemented. A lighter and inoculation loop are also pictured here.

In addition to common media preparations there are also some commercially prepared kits which are often used in clinical veterinary practices. Two such kits are Fungassay® **(Figure 12-3)** and Enerotube II® **(Figure 12-4)**. These are specialized media kits that are used frequently for diagnosis of ringworm (Fungassay®) and enterobacteria as well as Gram negative rod bacteria (Enerotube II®).

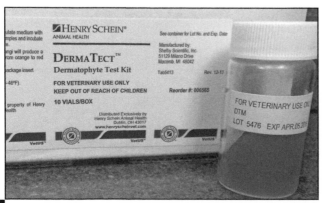

Figure 12-3: Fungal assay kits provide agar for growth of dermatophytes and may be purchased from a variety of sources. The slanted media is inoculated with suspect hair from areas suspect for dermatophytosis (ringworm). Picture courtesy of Holly Thomas.

The veterinary clinic which strives to create a small microbiological bench area will not generally have a need for a large variety of selective media and may wish to maintain media for only the most commonly seen microbial conditions. Each of the types of solid media may be poured in petri dishes and stored or in test tubes which may then be propped at a slanted angle to create "slants" as they solidify. Liquid media is placed in sterile tubes for best results and should never be used with petri dishes for liquid cultures due to awkwardness in handling and checking for results (swabs, etc.).

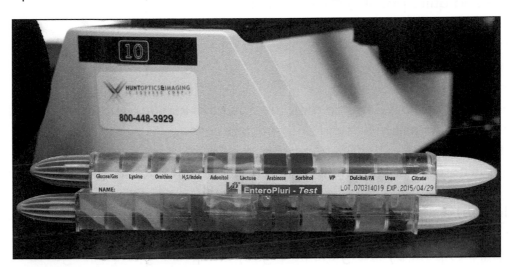

Figure 12-4: Enerotube® II is a rapid test system used to identify bacterial rods from the family Enterobacteriaceae. Each compartment contains different biochemical test which are needed to properly identify the bacteria. Picture courtesy of Holly Thomas.

## TABLE 12-1
### Commonly Used Media For Veterinary Microbiology Studies

| MEDIA | COMPONENTS | USAGE |
|---|---|---|
| Blood-Based Agar (S) | Trypticase soy agar, distilled water, defibrinated sheep/rabbit blood | Fastidious, pathogenic organisms |
| Enerotube II® (S) | Glucose, cresol red, lysine, bromocresol purple, ornithine, wax, sodium thiosulfate, ferric ammonium, citrate, tryptophan, adonitol, lactose, arabinose, sorbitol, urea, phenol red, sodium citrate, bromothymol blue. | Enteric pathogens |
| Fungassay® (S) | Soybean meal, dextrose phenol red, cycloheximide agar | *Microsporum canis* (ringworm) |
| Nutrient Agar (S) | Beef extract, peptone, agar | Basic microbiological usage |
| Nutrient Broth (L) | Beef extract, peptone | Basic microbiological usage |
| Nutrient gelatin (S) | Beef extract, peptone, gelatin | Basic microbiological usage |
| Staphylococcus media (S) | Yeast extract, tryptone, gelatin, lactose, d-Mannitol, sodium chloride dipotassium phosphate, agar | Suspect *Staphylococcus* sp infections |

Table 12-1: The following media are recommended for general purposes as clinics may wish to send less common case specimens to an outside facility for interpretation by a veterinary microbiologist or pathologist [(S): solid; (L): liquid].

# Media Preparation
## Dehydrated Media:

Due to the number of commercial suppliers who sell a variety of dehydrated media, it is recommended (if utilizing dehydrated media) to simply follow the manufacturer's instructions for best results. It is important to accurately measure all media and added liquid. Any deviations will cause erroneous results and quite possibly unusable media.

## Petri Dish (solid media): (1-125 mL bottle = 4 to 5 petri dishes):
1. Prepare a boiling water bath.*
2. Loosen the cap of the agar bottle.
3. Set the bottle in the boiling water to melt the agar, this may take up to 30 minutes.
4. Use an oven mitt to occasionally swirl and check progress.
5. Wipe down the work area with 70% alcohol or a 1:4 bleach/water mixture.
6. Once the agar is completely liquefied, carefully remove the bottle from the water and set it aside to cool slightly for 15 minutes** (the agar will not re-solidify).
7. Lay out sterile petri dishes that have been pre-labeled with Sharpie marker on bottom half of dish.
8. Remove the lid and wipe the rim of the bottle with an alcohol pad or flame it over a Bunsen burner and prepare to pour by lifting the lid slightly and pouring enough agar to cover only the bottom of the petri dish. Once poured, cover with a lid and set it aside.
9. Once plates are completely cooled and solid (approximately 30 minutes), they may be refrigerated upside down to avoid condensation and contamination of agar with moisture.

*A microwave may be useful in melting agar but must be done with cap removed and a piece of gauze placed over the opening and heating done in increments of 30 seconds to avoid overheating and spilling. Caution should be used in removing from microwave and oven mitt is recommended. Once melted begin at # 6 above.
**If poured while the agar is boiling or extremely hot, condensation is likely to occur as well as cracking of the agar once solidified.

## Tube Slants (solid media): (1-125 mL bottle = 25 tube slants of 5 mL media cultures):
1. Prepare a boiling water bath.*
2. Loosen cap of the agar bottle.
3. Set the bottle in boiling water to melt, this may take up to 30 minutes.
4. Use an oven mitt to occasionally swirl and check progress.
5. Wipe down the work area with 70% alcohol or 1:4 bleach/water mixture.
6. Once the agar is completely liquefied, carefully remove it from the water and set aside to cool slightly for 15 minutes** (the agar will not re-solidify).
7. Place sterile tubes that have been pre-labeled in a tube rack that can be autoclaved.
8. Using a sterile pipette or syringe, transfer 5 mL of melted agar into each tube.
9. Place caps loosely on the tubes and move them into an autoclave.
10. Autoclave at 250° Fahrenheit for 25 minutes.
11. Remove the tubes from the autoclave and tilt them slightly so that the cooling gel will form at a slanted angle.
12. Once cool, tighten the tube lids and refrigerate them for usage.

*A microwave may be useful in melting agar but must be done with cap removed and a piece of gauze placed over the opening and heating done in increments of 30 seconds to avoid over-heating and spilling. Caution should be used in removing from microwave and oven mitt is recommended. Once melted begin at # 6 above.

**If poured while the agar is boiling or extremely hot, condensation is likely to occur as well as cracking of the agar once solidified.

## Nutrient Broth (1-125 ml bottle of broth = 25 tubes of 5 ml broth cultures):

1. Wipe down the work area with 70% alcohol or a 1:4 bleach/water mixture.
2. Place sterile tubes that have been pre-labeled in a tube rack that can be autoclaved.
3. Using a sterile pipette or syringe after wiping the lip of the bottle, transfer 5 mL of liquid agar into each tube.
4. Autoclave the tubes at 250° Fahrenheit for 25 minutes.
5. Remove the tubes from the autoclave and allow them to cool completely before tightening the lids and refrigerating them for later use.

## Commercial Agar Kits:

The three most common agars that may be purchased ready-to-use are Enterotube II (Becton-Dickinson), Fungassay (Zoetis) and prepared plates, slants and broths from companies such as Carolina Biological and NASCO. These kits must be stored according to the manufacturer's directions, with most requiring refrigeration for preservation until used. Failure to handle and store the kits at proper temperatures may yield erroneous results which cannot be relied upon diagnostically. It is important to note the expiration date clearly on box or storage container so that the oldest may be used first to avoid waste. All expired media should be discarded. All expired media should be discarded.

# Laboratory Session – Microbiological Preparation

The purpose of this lab is to prepare plates, slants and broth tubes which may be used in Labs 13 and 14. The agar media which will be used is bottled media.

## Supplies Needed Per Group of 3 Students:

(2) 125 ml bottles of nutrient broth agar gel.
(1) 125 ml bottle of nutrient broth.
5 to 6 petri dishes.
8 to 10 glass test tubes.
Pipettes or 10 mL syringes (sterile).
Alcohol pads OR Bunsen burner.
70% alcohol OR bleach/water mix of 1:4 ratio.
Disposable towels.

## Supplies Needed for the Entire Class (set up as a centralized station):

√ Hot water bath or microwave.
√ Autoclave.

## Instructions:

1. After breaking into groups of 2 to 3 students, clean work areas with 70% alcohol (or a bleach/water mix).

2. Label the bottoms of the petri dishes with a group number, agar type and the date poured. (Example: GRP 1/NBA/DP: 6-1-2021).

3. Label the tubes for agar slants in the same fashion as the petri dishes.

4. Label the tubes for the broth (Example: GRP 1/NB/DP: 6-1-2021).

5. Refer to the instructions for creating agar plates, slants and tubes and begin to work.

6. Once prepared, these plates and tubes must be allowed to cool completely before storing in an appropriate fashion in the lab refrigerator for use in Labs 13 and 14.

7. Clean the area before leaving the lab by wiping down with either 70% Alcohol or bleach and water mixed in a 1:4 ratio.

# REFERENCES

1. Brown, A. E. (2012). Benson's Microbial Applications: Laboratory Manual in General Microbiology (Complete Version). New York, NY: McGraw-Hill Company.

2. NA. (2007, January). Becton-Dickinson. Retrieved from BD-BBL Enterotube II Instructions for Use: https://legacy.bd.com/europe/regulatory/Assets/IFU/HB/CE/ETUT/IA-273176.pdf

3. Quinn, P., Markley, B., Leonard, F., FitzPatrick, E., Fanning, S., & Hartien, P. (2011). Veterinary Microbiology and Microbial Disease, 2nd Edition. Ames, Iowa: Wiley-Blackwell.

4. Studdert, V. G. (2012). SaundersComprehensive Veterinary Dictionary, 4th Edition. New York, New York: Elsevier-Saunders.

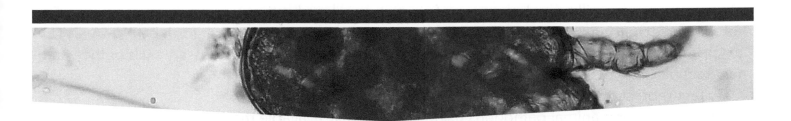

# CHAPTER 13

## MICROBIOLOGICAL SUPPLIES AND COLLECTION OF VETERINARY SPECIMENS

# OBJECTIVES

This lab addresses a variety of microbiological methodologies which may be encountered both in the clinical veterinary practice and within a veterinary clinical laboratory. The main focus of this laboratory exercise will be to become proficient at sample collection, preparation and plating. The Veterinary Technician Student Essential and Recommended Skills List as set forth by AVMA-CVTEA in Appendix I; Section 6 – Laboratory Procedures lists the following as necessary skills of the veterinary technician.

√ Collect representative samples
√ Identify common animal pathogens using commercially available media and reagents
√ Perform common biochemical tests
√ Perform staining procedures

# KEY TERMS

Aerobic

Anaerobic

Biological Wastes

Contamination

Culturettes®

Exudate

Hyperthermophiles

Mesophiles

Prions

Psychrophiles

Sterility

Thermophiles

# INTRODUCTION

Microbiology is firmly rooted within veterinary science as the study of microbial pathogens and infectious disease as it applies to animals and in some cases the humans who come into contact with them. From the earliest discoveries by Koch of *Bacillus anthracis* in the blood of animals which died from anthrax to the discovery of prions in the late 20th Century and the current scientific breakthroughs regarding the Covid-19 pandemic - microbiological investigations have played an important role in diagnostic veterinary medicine.

# DISCUSSION

The most effective microbiological-assisted diagnoses begin with the successful and aseptic isolation and collection of sample material. The samples may present from various areas of the body; each with specific collection and handling protocols which must be observed. Because microbiology involves the collection of organisms which will then be cultured on an appropriate growth media for identification, it is imperative to practice aseptic technique. Improper or casual collection of samples may allow for contamination with outside organisms or other debris which could lead to confusion and misdiagnosis.

Proper collection begins with access to the site of interest and having the appropriate vessels for collection and immediate preservation of the sample. Among the most common specimens collected in veterinary medicine are sputum, nasal and other respiratory discharge, tracheal wash contents, skin scrapings, wound exudate, vaginal discharge and ear exudate. It is also possible to culture blood and urine however the subject of culture and sensitivity testing will be covered in Lab 14.

To collect specimens from any of the areas mentioned above, you must not disturb the natural condition that is present in the area prior to collection. For instance, if a wound is not healing, has an odd odor and copious discharge, do not clean the area you intend to sample by performing a surgical scrub prior to sampling the exudate. Collection and subsequent culturing of the specimen will not be accurate because the wound was sanitized before collection.

The devices and supplies that are utilized for culturing a wound should also be sterile when they are used. Sterility of collection tools is the only way to assure that the sample collected is "pure" and not contaminated by outside sources. For this reason, it is suggested that only sterile, pre-packaged devices be utilized such as Culturettes® or sterile syringes. Once these items are used, they should be regarded as biological wastes and dealt with accordingly.

Once a specimen is collected, it must be properly preserved to avoid contamination and breakdown of specimen integrity. This includes determining if the organisms in the sample are aerobic or anaerobic to adequately provide for their continued survival. The need or lack of need for oxygen is the first diagnostic clue to microbial identification. Once a sample is collected, it should be sealed in a sterile container/environment for transport to the laboratory as quickly as possible.

Specimens should also be protected against temperature changes and light during transport. The temperature that a collected specimen is exposed to during transport can directly affect surviv-ability; temperature can also influence overgrowth of bacteria within the sample which in turn may affect diagnostic quality and outcome. There are four recognized groups of bacteria (psychro-philes, mesophiles, thermophiles and hyperthermophiles) but only one is of direct importance to the veterinary technician. The majority of pathogenic bacteria are "mesophiles" which survive and exhibit optimal growth between 20° and 45°C (68 and 113°F). Many of the pathogenic bacteria which may cause illnesses in animals may also spread disease in human populations (i.e. zoonoses). **Table 13-1** is a quick reference guide for veterinary technician students striving to understand the microbes of veterinary importance.

# CONCLUSION

The veterinary technician who understands the process of microbiological collection, preparation and interpretation is worth his/her weight in gold. Without an understanding of aseptic technique and the avoidance of contamination it is impossible and fruitless to attempt to identify microbes which may be causing illness. Although the microbes which have been identified in veterinary medicine do not generally change at an alarming rate, the methodologies and tools of the trade do improve continuously. It therefore behooves the technician with a keen interest in veterinary microbiology to continue to update their knowledge through CE opportunities as well as wet labs that may be offered at conference and convention venues.

## TABLE 13-1
## Veterinary Microbes*

| MICROBES | GRAM STATUS | HABITATS | ASSOCIATED ANIMAL HOST |
|---|---|---|---|
| Micrococcus luteus | + cocci (pairs) | Mammalian skin | Various mammals |
| Staphylococcus epidermis | + cocci (pairs/tetrads) | Mammalian skin | Various mammals |
| Staphylococcus agalactiae | + cocci (chains) | Vaginal/respiratory tract | Cattle |
| Streptococcus bovis | + cocci (pairs/chains) | Alimentary canal | Cattle, sheep and pigs |
| Streptococcus dysagalactiae | + cocci (chains) | Mammary glands | Cattle |
| Streptococci equi | + cocci (pairs/chains) | Respiratory system and lymph nodes | Equine |
| Rhodococcus equi | + cocci/+rods | Respiratory system | Foal |
| Corynebacterium sp. | + pleomorphic | Mammary glands | Cattle |
| Streptococcus sp. | + cocci (chains) | Mammary glands | Variety of animals |
| Staphylococcus sp. | + cocci (clusters) | Skin | Mammals |
| Listeria sp. | + rods | Respiratory system, oral, central nervous system, tonsils, soil, carcasses Alimentary canal | Domestic and wild animals Pigs and turkeys Mammals Mammals and birds |
| Erysipelothrix Bacillus anthracis Clostridium sp. | + rod or filament + rods + rods | Mixed locations | Many classes of animals affected. |

Source: Veterinary Microbiology and Microbial Disease

*This is a partial listing of some of the most common pathogenic microbes seen in veterinary medicine. For a more complete listing, consult textbooks or reference manuals devoted to veterinary microbiology.

# LABORATORY SESSION

# INSTRUCTIONS

Based on availability of specimens, your instructor will advise you regarding the collection and plating of specimens. You will be utilizing the microbiological growth media prepared during the last lab.

## Collection Techniques:

**a. Collection of Wound Exudate (possible infection)**

   i. Supplies:

      1. Culturette® tubes **(Figure 13-1)**

      2. Blood-based agar plates **(Figure 13-2)**

      3. Incubator **(Figure 13-3)**

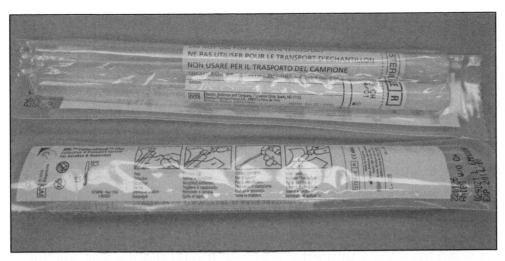

Figure 13-1: Culturette® tubes are commercially available and contain sterile microbial collection swabs. These swabs make sterile tissue or fluid collection easy and are a vital part of clinical practice.

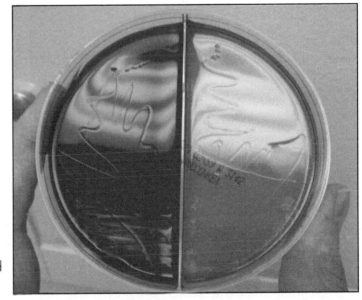

Figure 13-2: Blood-based agar plates are the cornerstone for bacterial cultures. Labs that perform routine microbiologic cultures will carry blood-based agar plates at a minimum. The plate featured has both blood (left) and MacConkey (right) agar halves.

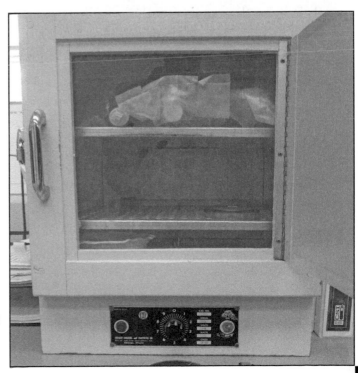

Figure 13-3: Incubators come in many varieties and (if working properly) maintain a specific temperature and environment appropriate for the microbial growth being studied. Small bench top incubators, such as featured here, are common in private veterinary practice.

ii. Instructions
   1. Identify the wound and ascertain the best method of restraining the animal.
   2. If hair is present, either clip it away from the wound or smooth it away from the wound for ease of access. Do not wet or apply any liquid to hair when smoothing away from collection area.
   3. Unwrap the Culturette® and remove the swab taking care not to touch the rayon tip to any surface.
   4. Swab the middle area of the wound in an attempt to collect as much exudate as possible.
   5. Withdraw the swab and replace it in the Culturette® media. Label it with the patient name, time collected, and areas collected from (i.e. vagina, wound, nasal, etc.).
   6. Upon return to the laboratory, label the bottom of the petri dish containing blood-based agar with the patient name, date and sample collected.
   7. Remove the swab from the Culturette® and with the lid slightly ajar, roll the swab over the media taking care not to break the surface of the media (no gouging). Refer to the diagrams below for swabbing direction.
   8. Incubate for 48 hours at 40°C.

b. **Collection of Ear Exudate (possible ear mites or yeast infection).**
   i. Supplies
      1. Ear swabs (sterile) or Culturettes®
      2. Microscope slides
      3. Lactophenyl Cotton Blue Stain or Methylene Blue stain
      4. Oil
      5. Sharpie marker
   ii. Instructions
      1. Lay out 2 microscope slides and label with the animal name and date, and number each slide (Left and Right).
      2. Restrain the animal firmly and advance the swab into the outer ear to collect visible exudate. Do not stick the swab deep into the ear canal where it is not visible.
      3. Rotate the swab gently to collect exudate and withdraw the swab. Repeat the process using a new swab in the other ear.
      4. On microscope slide Left place a drop of mineral oil and rotate the first swab to cover the slide with exudate and set the slide aside.
      5. On microscope slide Right roll the second swab to cover the slide with exudate.
      6. Place 1 drop of Lactophenol Cotton Blue or Methylene Blue stain on the exudate and mix it with a sterile toothpick before placing a coverslip over the sample.
      7. View each slide under the microscope (hi-Dry). **Figure 13-4** provides identification of ear mites (Otodectes spp). **Figure 13-5** provides identification of aural yeast (Malassezia pachydermatis) commonly associated with otitis externa.
      8. To culture and confirm fungi such as *M. pachhydermatis*, exudate from the skin or ears should be plated on prepared, blood based agar or McConkey Agar plates before incubating for 48 hours at 40°C or 37°C for 3 to 4 days on Sabouraud Dextrose agar.

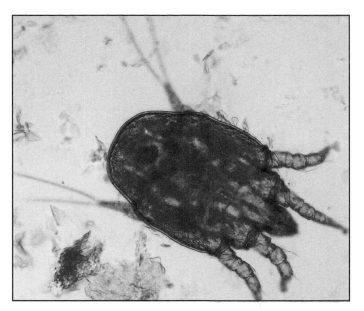

Figure 13-4: Ear mites (*Otodectes sp.*) are common infectious ear parasites of dogs and cats.

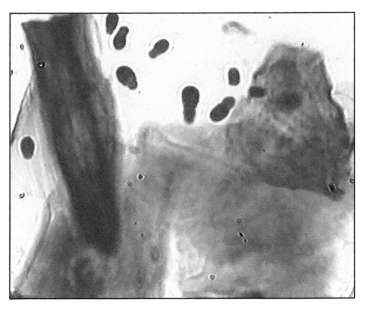

Figure 13-5: Classic *Malassezia pachydermatis* budding yeast are seen on a modified Wright's stain slide of dog ear exudate (100x). Ear cytology is necessary to make a microscopic diagnosis of yeast otitis externa.

## c. Slide Creation:

i. Supplies:
1. Microscope slides
2. Forceps or wooden clothe-pins
3. Petri dish (incubated x 48 hours)
4. Bunsen burner
5. Inoculating needle or loop
6. Water
7. Sharpie® marker

ii. Instructions:
1. Draw a circle approximately the size of a quarter with the sharpie marker on a microscope slide.
2. Flame the loop, then use the sterilized loop to place 2 loops full of water inside of the circle.
3. Flame the loop and set it aside **(Figure 13-6)**
4. Open the top of the petri dish just enough for the loop to pass through, flame the loop to sanitize and then pass it over the top of the media in the petri dish taking care not to gouge the media **(Figure 13-7)** Scrape a sample of the growth from the surface and withdraw the loop.
5. Smear the sample inside the circle on the microscope slide, mixing the sample with the water.
6. Flame the loop to sanitize and set it aside.
7. Attach a clothespin, or forceps to the microscope slide and wave it over the flame of the Bunsen burner, this will kill the bacteria in the specimen and fix it to the slide for staining.
8. Allow the slide to cool.

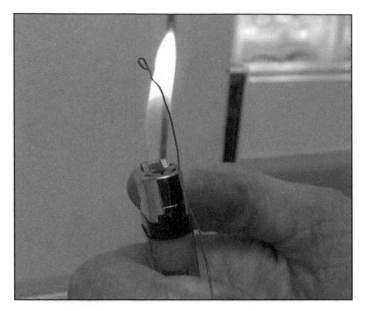

Figure 13-6: Culture loops are best sterilized by 'flaming' with a lighter or other lab safe fire or intense heat source. The end of the loop should turn bright red-yellow to ensure that the metal is hot enough to destroy any micro-organisms present.

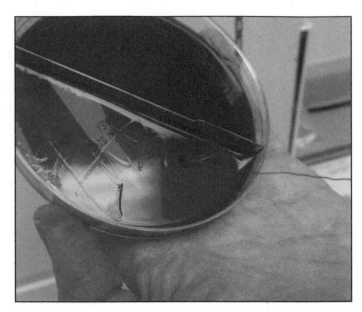

Figure 13-7: Culture loops can easily damage culture media. When plating organisms, carefully pass the culture loop over the media being careful to not create tears. This process is called 'streaking' or 'streaking the plate'.

## d. Staining Procedures: Gram Stain

i. Supplies:
1. Crystal Violet (primary stain)
2. Gram's Iodine (mordant)
3. Acetone (decolorizer)
4. Safranin
5. Water in a squirt bottle
6. Bibulous paper

ii. Instructions:
1. Cover a slide with Crystal Violet and let it stand for 20 seconds **(Figure 13-8)**.
2. Wash the slide with water for 2 to 5 seconds.
3. Cover the slide with Gram's Iodine and let it stand for 1 minute.
4. Rinse the slide gently with acetone (decolorizer) for approximately 10 to 20 seconds or until the acetone runs clear.
5. Wash the slide with water for 2 to 5 seconds.
6. Cover the slide with Safranin and let it stand for 1 minute.
7. Wash the slide with water for 2 to 5 seconds.
8. Blot the slide with bibulous paper and allow it to dry before looking at it under the microscope.

iii. Interpretation:
1. Purple cells: Gram positive (+) **(Figure 13-9)**.
2. Pink-reddish cells: Gram negative (-).
3. Rods = baccilli.
4. Round = cocci.

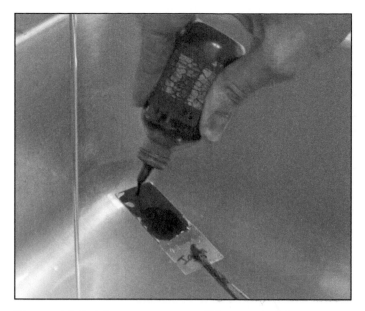

Figure 13-8: There are many different staining methods available. Each one has advantages and disadvantages. Regardless, be sure to follow staining instructions as directed by the manufacturer. Also follow reported safety guidelines as many stains use toxic compounds that require special handling.

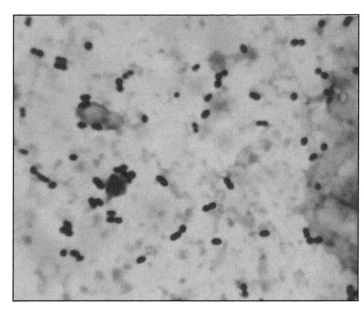

Figure 13-9: Gram stain of an ear swab in a dog. Gram positive (purple) paired cocci dominate the slide.

5. Multi-shape = pleomorphic.
6. Spiral = spirillum or spiroform.
7. Corkscrew = spirochetes.

# CONCLUSION

Complete the lab exercises above then utilize the knowledge and experience which you have gained to complete the worksheet.

# LAB 13: WORKSHEET

Name/Group Name: _____

Date:_____

## Wound Culture

Patient ID: _____

Species/Breed: _____

Sex:_____

History of Wound (cause, time wounded, Rx to date):_____

_____

Appearance of Wound (odor, drainage, etc.):_____

_____

Area Cultured (area of body, orifice, etc. – be descriptive in your answer):_____

_____

Collection Method for Wound Exudate:_____

Means of Preservation (Culturette, slide, etc.):_____

Plated/Incubated on (date/time):_____

Type of Pattern Used in Plating:_____

Gram Stain/Read on (date/time):_____

Findings (type of bacteria, Gram results, etc.):_____

_____

Draw the appearance of the bacteria in the circle below, indicate with colored pencils if organisms are Gram + or Gram -.

# Ear Exudate

Patient ID: _____

Species/Breed: _____

Sex: _____

Slide # 1 Stain Used: _____

Slide # 1 Result: _____

Slide # 2 Stain Used: _____

Slide # 2 Results: _____

Draw in the circles below the appearance of organisms as seen on examination of the microscope slides.

Questions and Answer (utilize your lab manual, textbook and other references to answer):

1. What would you consider to be the major difference between the four types of bacteria (RODS, COCCI, SPIROCHETE AND PLEOMORPHIC)? _____

_____

2. What reason would you give to a client who asked why you were taking a sample of the wound exudate on their pet?_____

3. You are on a farm call with your veterinarian and he decides to take a swabbed culture from the family dog that has a nasty laceration from a run-in with a barb-wire fence. He sends you back to the truck to retrieve supplies to do this, what do you bring him and why (assume the truck is really decked out with everything you can think of)?_____

_____

4. You have now assisted in culturing the dog's wound in # 3, how do you transport this back to the lab, it is 90 degrees in the shade and the date is August 15th, again you have lots of things in the truck to choose from:_____

_____

5. You arrive back at the lab, what are you going to plate the wound exudate on and why:_____

_____

6. How long does this have to incubate and at what temperature: _____

_____

7. The veterinarian prefers to read all Gram stains himself, however after he does, he calls you over, inviting you to see the *Staphylococcus epidermis*. What should you expect to see on this slide:_____

_____

8. Based on the findings of #7 is this the cause of the purulent discharge in the wound, why or why not?_____

_____

9. What are nosocomial infections, why are they important within the medical community (both human and veterinary)? _____

_____

10. Is MRSA a concern in veterinary medicine, why or why not?_____

_____

# REFERENCES

1. Brown, A. E. (2012). Benson's Microbial Applications: Laboratory Manual in General Microbiology (Complete Version). New York, NY: McGraw-Hill Company.
2. Hendrix, C., & Sirois, M. (2007). Laboratory Procedures for Veterinary Technicians. St. Louis: Mosby-Elsevier.
3. Meyer, D. A. (2004). Veterinary Laboratory Medicine - Interpretation and Diagnosis, 3rd Ed. St. Louis: Saunders.

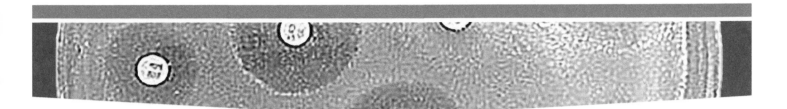

# CHAPTER 14

## MICROBIAL CULTURE AND SENSITIVITY AND BIOCHEMICAL TESTING

# OBJECTIVES

This laboratory addresses the following Veterinary Technician Student Essential and Recommended Skills List as set forth by the AVMA-CVTEA in Appendix I, Section 6: Laboratory Procedures.

√ Culture bacteria and perform sensitivity tests
√ Culture and identification of common dermatophytes
√ Identify common animal pathogens using commercially available media and reagents
√ Perform common biochemical tests

# KEY TERMS

| | | |
|---|---|---|
| Adonitol | Dermatophyte | Ornithine Decarboxylase |
| Aerobic | Dulcitol | Phenylalanine Deaminase |
| Anaerobic | Glucose | Reagents |
| Antimicrobials | Indole | Sensitivity |
| Arabinose | Inoculation | Sorbitol |
| Aspiration | Kovac's Reagent | Sulfonamides |
| Broth | Lactose Decarboxylase | Tetracycline |
| Citrate | Lysine | Urea |
| Culture | Media | Voges-Proskauer Test |

# INTRODUCTION

The veterinary technician who is well versed in the use of microbiological culturing techniques as a way of identifying pathogens and determining sensitivity to proposed treatment plans is an invaluable asset to a clinician. The introduction of the supplies needed to establish an in-house "micro lab" is inexpensive and need not take up a large amount of space.

Additionally, the use of microbiological testing in-house may hasten results and add to the revenue potential of the clinic. Technicians should also be familiar with the various types of reagents as well as biochemical testing kits/methods which are available for quick point-of-care testing. Consider monitoring expiration dates to be a top priority. Expired reagents, test kits and agar kits may lead to erroneous results and should be discarded immediately according to manufacturer instructions.

# SAFETY NOTICE

As with handling any animal tissue, special care should be taken with microbial samples. Most microbial organisms are not dangerous and are handled by a normally functioning immune system in both animals and humans. However, some organisms are pathogenic, multi-drug resistant and/or zoonotic. Higher than average concentrations of potentially dangerous microbial organisms are encountered in hospitals, research facilities and other locations where sick animals are handled. A successful culture further concentrates microbial organisms creating greater risk of exposure, even if accidental.

The Centers for Disease Control and Prevention has created Biosafety Levels (BSL's) 1 to 4 based on the potential danger of the microbe in question. A quick review of the different BSL's can be found at https://www.cdc.gov/cpr/infographics/biosafety.htm.

If the veterinary technician has an immune system disorder, takes immune suppressive drugs, chemo-therapy or is otherwise at greater risk for contracting an infectious disease, discuss with your instructor prior to handling any microbial agents. Otherwise, practice safe handling, use of personal protective equipment and wash hands thoroughly after working with any potentially infectious agents.

# DISCUSSION

There are a variety of methods which may be utilized for determining the presence of pathological microbes as well as some parasites. This lab will explore some of the most commonly encountered laboratory tests regarding culture and sensitivity as well as pathogen identification. When dealing with microbiological diagnostics, the majority of procedures require periods of incubation before identification as well as assessment of antimicrobial sensitivity. As reviewed in Chapter 13, it is imperative to practice strict, aseptic technique regarding the collection of samples and inoculation of media plates, tubes or broth; anything less can result in contamination and erroneous results. Erroneous results can then cause misdiagnosis and non-productive treatment.

# CULTURE METHODS AND MEDIA

The type of culture medium chosen is partly dependent on the site of sampling. Some of the considerations that should be taken into account when choosing culture media include:

√ Is the sample from an aerobic or anaerobic site?
√ What is the nature of the collection environment (i.e. moist/dry; internal/external; blood based)?

To facilitate successful collection of microbial life for incubation, sterile instruments must be used to avoid additional contamination of the sample and to prevent destruction of collected microbial life or further contamination of the site. To aid in the provision and maintenance of an aseptic environment during collection (and later inoculation) there are several inexpensive, commercial collection devices such as scalpel blades, swabs (both cotton and rayon), plastic inoculation loops and wires available. For the cost-conscious individual, it is acceptable to pre-sterilize existing equipment such as metal loops and wires, forceps or scalpels. It is up to the individual facility to decide which is best for their clinic based on the estimated number of cases which are seen requiring microbiological diagnoses. Both have their advantages and disadvantages with cost not necessarily being the deciding factor for usage.

The collection of microbiological specimens may be done by swabbing (preferably using Rayon swabs or Culturettes®), scraping (utilizing scalpels) squash prep or aspiration (using a needle and syringe). The instruments used for such techniques are all commonly found in the clinical setting. The key to success is sterility and aseptic technique during collection. The sample should be collected from the most active area of the lesion or wound to increase the chances of retrieving a large number of organisms. Sometimes microbial samples must be taken from the "environment" that the suspected pathogen normally inhabits. This is the case with samples such as milk or urine specimens which should be handled aseptically.

The growth media which is chosen for a particular culture must reflect a similar environment as that from which the sample was originally collected. The selected media provides nutrients, proper $O_2$

requirements (or lack thereof in the case of anaerobic bacteria) and an environment conducive to optimal growth of the organism for later identification.

It is important to understand and utilize the proper agar (i.e. growth media) in order to facilitate microbial growth. The various media are available either as dehydrated bulk media to be prepared as needed or commercially prepared media plates, slants and broth for immediate usage with little or no preparation required. It is recommended that you follow the manufacturer's directions to create a suitable environment for the suspected organisms if dehydrated media is used.

## CONCLUSION

The use of microbiology in veterinary diagnostics is an invaluable tool which can yield quick results and boost the economic growth of a practice if implemented by individuals with a knowledge, appreciation and interest in the field. Veterinary technicians are such individuals because their training allows them to understand the need for precise, clinical collection of samples and also provides a good basic understanding of the various methods of microbiological testing displaying skill at the microbiology bench.

# LABORATORY SESSION

## INSTRUCTIONS

Complete the diagnostic testing outlined within this lab and note the results on the laboratory worksheet. This laboratory assignment will require two lab sessions (or visits to the lab) to complete since many of the cultures must incubate for 24 to 48 hours. Where commercial kits are provided, consult the manufacturer's instructions (due to possible changes/updates that supersede the laboratory manual) in addition to the lab manual for best results.

To complete each culturing exercise, the following supplies are needed per group of 2 students, the number in parentheses indicates the quantity of the item that is needed per group. The kits may differ according to availability in your program. Your instructor will provide instructions if the kits differ.

√ Flexicult Urine Culture Plates (Atlantic Diagnostics) (1).
√ BBL Enterotube II® (1), Enterotube Codebook (to be shared by class), Enterotube results sheet (1) (Bectin-Dickenson).
√ 3 ml of urine specimen (Figure 14-1).
√ Specimen on Mueller-Hinton plate of suspected enterobacterial microbes (48 hours or less in age) (1).
√ Sterile pipette (for urine transfer) (1).
√ Antibiotic sensitivity tests (multiple discs) (Figure 14-2).
√ Voges-Proskauer Reagent A and B.
√ Kovac's Reagent.

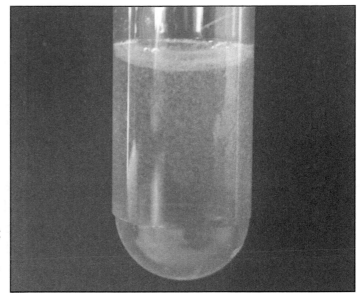

Figure 14-1: Collect urine using sterile methods such as cystocentesis. Other methods such as free catch or collection off a clean surface may also be acceptable but can be contaminated with organisms that are not truly present in the urine. The method of collection should be considered when interpreting urine culture results.

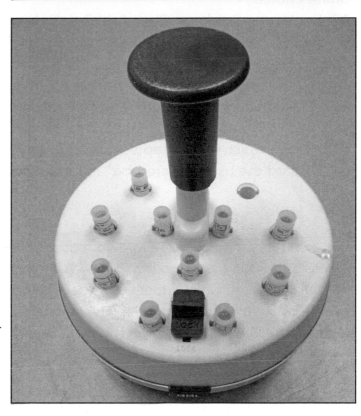

Figure 14-2: Antibiotic sensitivity disks are loaded into a specially designed dispenser. Dispensers are designed specifically to fit standard and some non-standard microbiologic growth medium (such as Mueller-Hinton) plates. The antibiotic sensitivity disks are distanced appropriately to provide the most meaningful results when completing a culture and sensitivity test.

# TO CULTURE USING ENTEROTUBE II®

1. Label the Enterotube® using a Sharpie marker with the patient name, date and group #.
2. Carefully remove the caps on both ends of the tube, do not touch the sterile wire under the white cap, do not flame or otherwise attempt to sterilize.
3. Identify isolated colonies on the previously inoculated plate and pick at the colony with the tip of the wire without touching the agar so that the inoculum can be seen on the tip and side of the wire.
4. Inoculate the Enterotube® by twisting and drawing the wire back through the 12 colored compartments of the Enterotube® and remove.
5. Reinsert the wire into the Enterotube® and through the previously inoculated compartments until the notch on the wire aligns itself with the tube opening. Break the wire at the notch.
6. With a broken wire, punch a small hole in the plastic covered air inlets of the following to provide

an aerobic environment: Adonitol, Lactose, Arabinose, Sorbitol, Voges-Proskauer, Dulcitol/PA, Urea and Citrate.

7. Incubate for 18 to 24 hours at 35 to 37°C. The tube may either rest on a flat surface or stand upright in a test tube rack within the incubator.

8. After 24 hours, remove the tube from the incubator to interpret and record all test results except those in the Indole and Voges-Proskauer testing area.

9. Reactions of all but Indole and Voges-Proskauer are read in sequence through color comparison. Positive results should be circled on the results sheet.

10. Next, use a hot needle or inoculating wire and melt a hole of 3 to 4 mm (diameter) in the plastic film over the Indole/$H_2$S and the Voges-Proskauer area.

11. For Indole/$H_2$S Test: Add 3 to 4 drops of Kovac's reagent to the Indole/$H_2$S compartment, ensuring that the reagent makes contact with the media. A positive reaction is the change of reagent color to red within 10 seconds. Indicate results on the results sheet by circling the appropriate choice.

12. For Voges-Proskauer Test: Add 3 to 5 drops of Voges-Proskauer reagent A and 1 to 2 drops of reagent B. Reaction may be read within 5 to 15 minutes (no more than 15), a positive reaction = cherry red color; a negative reaction = copper to brown color. Indicate the result on the chart by circling the appropriate choice on the results sheet.

13. Check the results chart for completeness, next add the circled numbers in each bracketed area and write the total in the squares. This 5-digit number represents a corresponding number in the code book which in turn represents an organism(s).

14. Discard the used Enterotube® in biohazard waste disposal units.

# TO CULTURE URINE

Urine cultures may be done for two reasons: to identify the pathogenic organisms present and to assess antibiotic susceptibility. This may be done by use of commercial kits such as Flexicult® Veterinary Urinary Test (which identifies certain pathogens as well as antibiotic resistance/susceptibility) or by direct examination of urine microscopically (see Chapter 3). Urine culturing is best accomplished by using fresh urine handled in the most aseptic manner possible regardless of the chosen technique.

# ANTIBIOTIC SUSCEPTIBILITY TESTING

It is possible to assess the susceptibility of plated microbial organisms to antibiotics through agar diffusion. To test an inoculated Mueller-Hinton plate, a selection of antibiotic discs that correspond to available antibiotics kept in-house for treatment purposes is needed (**Figures 14-3 and 14-4**). It is recommended that a selection of discs representing the tetracyclines and the sulfonamides should be placed on the surface of the agar. Take care to space the discs far enough apart so that they do not touch (approximately 10 mm) and guard against damaging the agar surface. Once the discs are in place, incubate them in an inverted position (to avoid condensation) at 37°C for 18 to 24 hours (overnight).

The method by which the discs are assessed is the presence of a zone of inhibition which is an observed diameter around the disc devoid of any microbial growth after 24 hours. This is most easily observed by looking through the underside of the plate and measuring with the use of calipers. The interpretation of this "zone of inhibition" as it relates to microbial susceptibility or

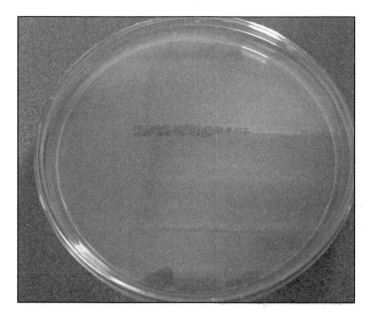

Figure 14-3: Mueller-Hinton plates are most commonly used for antibiotic sensitivity testing.

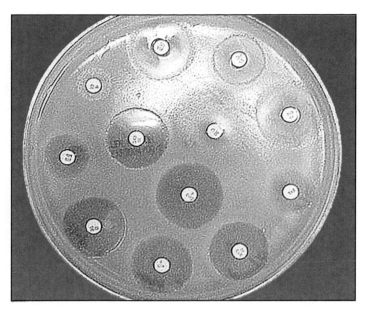

Figure 14-4: Mueller-Hinton plate inoculated with bacteria, with antibiotic sensitivity discs applied and then incubated. The 'zone of inhibition' (clear ring around each disc) is measured to determine how sensitive the organism is to each antibiotic found in the sensitivity discs.

resistance has been established by the National Committee for Clinical Laboratory Standards. A listing is also available at the following: https://clsi.org/standards/products/microbiology/documents/m52/.

# Culture of Dermatophytes

Similar to urine cultures, it is possible to culture dermatophytes for presence and treatment utilizing commercial culture sets (i.e. Fungassay®) or in-house agar plates (i.e. Sabouraud Dextrose Agar) which are efficient, inexpensive and easy to use. The optimal sample is broken or distorted hairs as well as crusted or scabbed over areas that fluoresce under a Wood's Lamp **(Figures 14-5 and 14-6)**. Hair is pressed into the media but not buried (agar should not be gouged or broken) before replacing the lid loosely to allow air exchange. It is not necessary to inoculate agar with large amounts of hair as this will cause overgrowth which will be useless diagnostically. Once inoculated, the labelled bottle is incubated at room temperature (72 to 86° F) for 48 hours before reading. The color change and growth observed on the media is considered a confirmatory test for dermatophytes. Precautions should be taken when handling the samples and test materials because dermatophytes are regarded as zoonotic in nature.

## Identification of Dermatophytes:

When culturing on Sabouraud-Dextrose agar, the appearance of the colonies will aid in differentiating the type of dermatophytes (i.e. fungi). Additionally, the shape of the fungi will further aid in identification when examined microscopically. **Table 14-1** provides a quick guide to common dermatophytes.

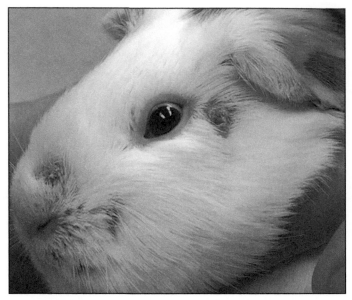

Figure 14-5: Guinea pig with ringworm (dermatophytosis). Skin lesions are often round areas of hair loss with varying degrees of skin scaling and redness. The round or 'ring' shaped lesion is in part why the disease is called 'ringworm'. However, this is a fungal and not worm-related parasitic disease. This guinea pig has suspicious skin lesions just caudal and ventral to the eye and on the side of the nose.

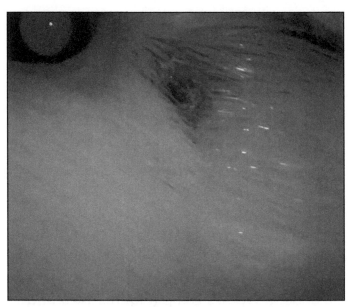

Figure 14-6: The same guinea pig as in the previous figure is fluoresced with a black light (Wood's lamp). The bright streaks are noted in the hairs around the skin lesion caudal and ventral to the eye. Some, but not all, dermatophytes will fluoresce under a black light giving a presumptive diagnosis of 'ringworm' or dermatophytosis. Culture, direct microscopic visualization and/or biochemical characterization are needed to definitively diagnose the organism.

## TABLE 14-1
## Dermatophyte Types

| DERMATOPHYTES | HOST(S) | APPEARANCE | COLONY APPEARANCE |
| --- | --- | --- | --- |
| Microsporum canis | Dog, cat | Spindle shape, thick walled | White, buff colored with orange periphery |
| Microsporum gypseum | Dog, horse, rodent | Boat shaped, thin walled | Buff-cinnamon colored with white border, powdery in appearance with the odor of rodent droppings present |
| Trichophyton mentagrophytes | Dog, horse, rodents, other species | Cigar shaped, thin walled | Creamy tan-buff colored, powdery |
| Trichophyton verrucosum (ringworm) | Cattle | Cocci-shaped chains | White color, velvety in heaps |

# LABORATORY 14 – WORKSHEET

1. Enterotube® Culture: Attach Enterotube® worksheet to laboratory submission. Complete the following:

Patient Name:_____ Sex:_____ Age:_____

Date Inoculated:_____

Date Read:_____

ID Value:_____

Organism ID:_____

2. Urine Culture: (using Flexicult)

Patient Name:_____ Sex:_____ Age:_____

Date Collected: _____

Collection Method: _____

Bacteria ID: _____

3. Antibiotic Susceptibility Testing (Kirby-Bauer):

Sample Used: _____ (patient/samples)

Inoculants: _____ (list all discs used)

Date Inoculated:_____

Date Read:_____

Inhibition Zone:_____ (record in millimeters, all disc areas displaying a clear zone)

4. Antibiotic Susceptibility: Indicate all displaying no growth (-) and growth (+)

_____Ampicillin

_____Amoxicillin/Clavulanate

_____Cephalothin

_____Enrofloxacin

_____Trimethoprim/Sulfamethoxazole

5. Dermatophyte Testing: for both commercial and in-house testing:

Patient Name:_____

Sample Site:_____

Date Inoculated:_____ (Fungassay)

Date Read:_____ (Fungassay)

Date Inoculated:_____ (Sabouraud-Dextrose)

Date Examined:_____ (Sabouraud-Dextrose)

Identification:_____

6. Please answer the following questions regarding the culture and sensitivity testing completed above:

A. From what site is the specimen collected that was tested using the Enterotube II®? What type of bacteria does this system identify?_____
_____

B. Name three common enterobacteria and explain their pathological importance. Are they considered zoonotic?_____
_____

C. Regarding the urine culture, provide a brief overview such as you would enter into the record regarding the patient's condition as well as results of the urine culture._____
_____
_____

D. What two types of susceptibility discs should be represented when performing the Kirby-Bauer technique? Why?_____
_____
_____

E. Name two common types of dermatophytes, describe their colony appearance on agar plates and discuss zoonotic implications._____
_____
_____

F. Discuss why aseptic technique is important in culturing exercises, name three areas of concern that may cause unexpected contamination._____

_____

_____

# REFERENCES

1. Brown, A. E. (2012). Benson's Microbial Applications, Complete Version, 12th Edition. New York, NY: McGraw-Hill.

2. Hendrix, C., & Sirois, M. (2007). Laboratory Procedures for Veterinary Technicians. St. Louis: Mosby-Elsevier.

3. NA. (2007, January). BD BBL Enterotube II. Retrieved on 9-6-2021 from: https://legacy.bd.com/europe/regulatory/Assets/IFU/HB/CE/ETUT/IA-273176.pdf

4. NA. (2013, December 13). Flexicult Vet Urinary Test. Retrieved on 9-6-2021 from: https://www.ssidiagnostica.com/flexicult-vet-urinary-test/

5. NA. (2013, December 31). Fungassay Dermatophyte Test Media. Retrieved on 9-6-2021 from: https://www2.zoetisus.com/products/diagnostics/referencelab/fungassay

6. Quinn, P., Markley, B., Leonard, F., FitzPatrick, E., Fanning, S., & Hartien, P. (2011). Veterinary Microbiology and Microbial Disease, 2nd Edition. Ames, Iowa: Wiley-Blackwell.

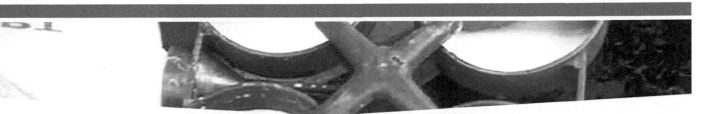

# CHAPTER 15

## MILK TESTING

# OBJECTIVES

This lab introduces the student to the methodologies involved in the testing of raw milk from large and small ruminant species. Although it is recognized that there are federal and state regulations in place for testing milk for human consumption, there is often a need as part of the diagnostic medical work-up for veterinarians to conduct point-of-care as well as laboratory testing in large animal species including small ruminant species.

This lab addresses the following Veterinary Technology Students Essential and Recommended Skills List as set forth by the AVMA-CVTEA in Appendix I, Section 6 – Laboratory Procedures:
√ Collect milk samples
√ Conduct mastitis testing (CMT, Culture)

# KEY TERMS

California Mastitis Testing (CMT)
CMT Reagent
ELISA
"First milk"

Johne's Disease
Mastitis
Non-Pasteurized
Pasteurized
PCR

Precipitate
Ruminants
Somatic Cell Count
Subclinical

# INTRODUCTION

While all mammals produce milk, the veterinary technician is most often required to test milk from ruminants – namely cattle, sheep and goats. The goat is responsible for supplying approximately 2% of the world's total supply of milk. The popularity of goat's milk has grown in the 21st Century due to its low fat percentage when compared to cow's milk. Cows continue however to produce the largest amount of milk consumed in the United States having produced 15.7 billion pounds of milk in December 2012 alone (per harvest from the US identified "23 major states" of production) (USDA, 2014) **(Figure 15-1)**. Healthy cows equal sellable milk and therefore large animal practitioners and associated veterinary technicians may find themselves performing milk testing often as part of a farm's herd health program or during emergency field calls.

# DISCUSSION

Milk testing may be performed by veterinary diagnostic laboratories through ELISA, PCR or other methods. This may be necessary when attempting to diagnose specific diseases such as Johne's disease. Some testing may also be carried out "cow-side" as a measure of point-of-care (POC) testing in the field. For the purpose of this laboratory activity, POC methods will be the focus.

Examination of milk may be required for a number of reasons including assessment of the quality of milk, bacterial load, and identification of specific pathogens such as _Salmonella, Streptococcus, Listeria_ or _Mycobacterium tuberculosis_. Mastitis, a common disease, is mostly seen in dairy goats and occasionally dairy cows and is generally spread by unsterile conditions involving the udder, teats, humans and milking parlor machinery. The most commonly encountered bacteria seen in mastitis cases are: _Staphylococcus epidermidis, Staphylococcus aureus,_ and _Streptococcus agalactiae._ Occasionally _E. Coli, Klebsiella, Pasteurella,_ and _Norcardia_ bacteria and _Candida_ yeast are seen. The

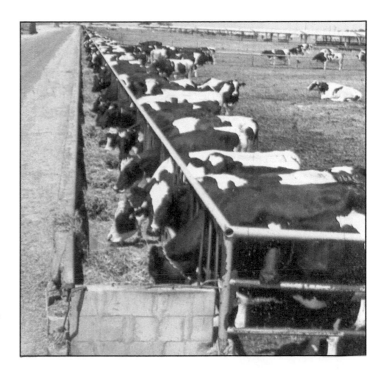

Figure 15-1: Cows dominate the milk market. However, goat and sheep milk represent a smaller but growing percentage of the market.

mode of infection involves microbes gaining access to the mammary gland and may be subclinical (no symptoms) or clinical (symptomatic) in nature and should be noted in the animal's records.

There are three main testing methods which are routinely conducted on fresh milk samples: microscopic examination of raw milk, milk cultures, and the California Mastitis Test (CMT) which assesses somatic cell counts. All tests are routinely performed in cases of suspected mastitis. While the CMT may be performed cow-side, the culturing of milk requires transportation back to the lab in a temperature controlled and aseptic manner; this includes keeping milk as cool (not frozen) as possible during transport. The culturing of milk may also be used to determine the sensitivity of microbes to available antibiotics as well as to determine antibiotic residue within milk samples (generally a public health concern of commercial milk companies buying large quantities for pasteurization and human consumption).

It is important to note that accurate sample collection and record keeping are mandatory because the milk industry involves public health and the livelihoods of the producers. Poor records and/or collection methods can ultimately result in unusable data, false positive or false negative results all of which may result in the milk being destroyed which has economic consequences to producers. These poor techniques can also potentially result in pathogenic organisms entering the human food chain resulting in a public health crisis that often requires local, state and national governmental intervention (i.e. government recalls, etc.). Having milk destroyed or the presence of infectious disease outbreaks related to the sale of milk products can have devastating effects on individual producers and the industry as a whole.

## Milk Collection:

Regardless of the method of testing when milk is collected, aseptic collection technique must be practiced in order to produce viable and diagnostically sound results. This also includes maintaining an aseptic environment for the collector (i.e. technician), the animal, and the milk itself to avoid contamination of the sample.

Animals should be restrained securely for ease of collection and the safety of both the human and the animal. This is generally accomplished by using large or small animal stocks or chutes. Never attempt to work with animal(s) without using proper restraint/safety equipment (ropes, harnesses, chutes, stocks). Once restrained, assess the level of cleanliness of the udder. If the udder is clean, wipe it with alcohol and allow it to air dry, if the udder is dirty and must be washed, use water to wash away grime before drying with single use towels and then wiping with alcohol and allowing it to air dry. Do not use soap and water and never attempt to "scrub" the udder, handle it gently **(Figure 15-2)**.

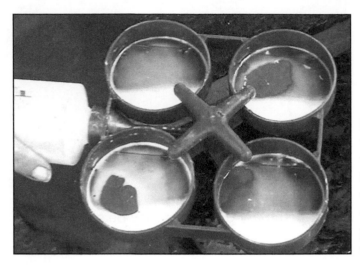

Figure 15-2: After the animal is appropriately restrained to prevent injury to people and the animal and prior to microbiologic sample collection, ensure the udder is clean. If dirty, gently wash and clean the udder with water (no deterngents or soap) and then wipe down with single use alcohol swabs and allow to air dry. Utilize paddles to collect milk from each of four quarters to ensure there is no cross contamination.

Next, using a cotton or rayon swab, swab the teat sphincter gently with alcohol before compressing the teat to express the "first milk" (generally 2 to 3 squirts of milk) which should be discarded. Now you are ready to collect the "sample" by squirting two to three squirts of milk into a collection vessel (sterile collection tube) before capping. Label as to which quarter the sample is collected from, also note in the records (Rockett & Bosted, 2007); for example:

L    Label    Example:    Records    Entry Example:   Milk sample collected 2/2/21 @
                                                      3 PM on cow # 310 from (list teat).

Cool but do not freeze the collected milk immediately using ice or ice packs in a cooler for transport to the laboratory. In the lab, inoculate plates or perform microscopic examination immediately. Never freeze a milk sample destined for testing or leave it at room temperature because the sample will be compromised. A milk sample should be tested as soon after arrival at the lab as possible for best results.

# LAB 15

## MATERIAL AND SUPPLIES

Alcohol
Antibiotic sensitivity discs
Blotting paper
Calipers or ruler
Catch basin
Colony counter

Distilled water
Forceps
Hot water bath loops
Incubator
Methylene Blue
Microscope

Microscopic slides
Milk
Mueller-Hinton agar plates
Nutrient agar plates
3 sterile bottles with 99 ml of
sterile water
Xylene

# INTRODUCTION

Milk testing is done for a variety of reasons but generally as a means of assessing not only the quality of raw milk but also as a means of identifying and assessing the types of pathogens that may be present. Aseptic technique during the collection, preservation and testing of the milk sample is critical.

This lab session will allow the student to become proficient in the methods of collection and testing raw milk samples: microscopic examination, standard colony plate counts and enumeration of cells, California Mastitis Test (CMT) and culturing and sensitivity testing for antibiotic usage. Refer to the earlier discussion on animal handling and restraint for collection of milk in order to collect samples for the lab. If time is critical, your instructor may provide previously collected milk for you to test.

# MATERIAL AND SUPPLIES

| | |
|---|---|
| CMT paddles | Restraint chute for cow |
| CMT reagent | Ruler |
| Cow | Towels |
| Gloves | Warm water |

## Instructions
### Microscopic Examination:

1. Spread .01 ml of milk over a clean microscope slide (this equates to a microbiological loop full of milk).
2. Allow the slide to air dry (do not flame).
3. Fix over the steam of a hot water bath for 5 minutes.
4. Cover the slide with xylene (known to be carcinogenic, wear gloves) and let it sit for 1 minute to remove all fat from the milk sample.
5. Wash the sample with alcohol to remove the xylene (capture the rinse material in a basin for disposal, do not pour it down the sink drain).
6. Wash the sample with distilled water to remove the alcohol (capture rinse material in a basin for disposal, do not pour it down sink drain).
7. Cover the sample with methylene blue for 15 seconds.
8. Rinse gently with water and blot dry for examination under the microscope.
9. Examine for bacteria and cells, enumerate and record results on the lab sheet (as well as the animal records if applicable).

### Enumeration of Cells:

To enumerate the cells seen in the milk sample, count and make note of the number of organisms in 3 to 5 separate fields over the entire area of the slide. Then take an average of these fields and report as "average per field" or "#APF". Next take this average and multiply it by the microscope factor (4x, 10x, etc.) that the slide was examined with to get a direct microscope count per ml of milk. This is reported as "Microbial count per mL". If the calculation is less than 500,000, the milk is considered of good bacteriological quality while 20,000,000 or more denotes milk of very poor quality to be discarded and not suitable for human consumption.

# Example of enumeration of a Count:

Field # 1  =  80
Field # 2  =  120
Field # 3  =  30
Field # 4  =  70
Field # 5  =  50
TOTAL        350/5 = 70
If counted using focal distance of 10x on microscope: 70 (10) = 700
If counted using focal distance of 4x on microscope: 70(4) = 280

# Milk Culture: (Standard Plate Count):

Before actually placing the milk on a microbiological culture plate to grow, the milk should be diluted in order to facilitate the determination of bacterial numbers. In order to do this, fill each of three sterile bottles with 99 mL of sterile water and label the bottles A, B and C.

Into Bottle A place 1 ml of the milk sample and cap, then shake vigorously for good distribution of the bacteria. Next using a new pipette, remove 1 ml of the milk from Bottle A, place it into Bottle B and shake vigorously. Finally using a fresh pipette, draw 1 ml of milk from Bottle B, add it to Bottle C and shake vigorously. These three bottles should have the following dilution factors:

Bottle A  =  1:100
Bottle B  =  1:10,000
Bottle C  =  1:1,000,000

Next, label the bottom of four previously poured nutrient agar plates as follows before plating aliquots as designated:

Inoculation Guidelines

| Plate | Labeled Nutrient Agar Plate | Add Sample |
|-------|-----------------------------|------------|
| 1 | Milk – 1:100,000 B | .1 ml of sample from Bottle B |
| 2 | Milk – 1:10,000 B | 1.0 ml of sample from Bottle B |
| 3 | Milk – 1:1,000,000 C | 1.0 ml of sample from Bottle C |
| 4 | Milk – 1:10,000,000 | .1 ml of sample from Bottle C |

Incubate the agar plates for 48 hours at 25°C before examining. Enumerate by counting the number of colonies present (this may be done with or without an electronic, lighted colony counter). The number reported is recorded as the "colony forming units" (CFU's) and represents live, viable cells. A sample yielding 30 to 300 CFU's is considered to be statistically relevant and valid. If a plate yields over 300 colonies, it should be regarded as "overgrown", less than 30 colonies indicates a sampling or plating error. All results should be recorded in the lab report and in the animal records if appropriate.

# Antibiotic Sensitivity:

An antibiotic disc can be used to assess whether or not a microbe is susceptible to a specific antibiotic treatment. To perform antibiotic susceptibility, sub-culturing is needed after the culture has produced colonies.

1. Using Bottle A from the Standard Plate Count lab above, plate a sample on to a Mueller-Hinton agar plate, label and incubate the plate for 48 hours.

2. Inoculate the Mueller-Hinton plate with a variety of antibiotic sensitivity discs. Be careful to only use one representative from the tetracyclines and one from the sulfonamides to prevent possible cross resistance. Be sure to place the discs far enough apart to avoid confusion regarding the antibiotic susceptibility. It is recommended to visualize the agar plate as the face of a clock and place the discs at 12, 3, 6 and 9 o'clock staying approximately 15 mm from the edge of the plate (please refer to **Figure 14-4**). The green circles represent the antibiotic disc; the orange circles represent zones of inhibition that surround the discs. If there is no orange zone, the disc is not effective against the bacteria.

3. Incubate the plate aerobically at 37°C for 18 to 24 hours before observing for "zone of inhibition".

4. To assess zone of inhibition, read at 18 to 24 hours by using a clear ruler or calipers to measure on the underside of the plate. The measurement should include both the diameter of the disc as well as the area cleared of growth (zone of inhibition). Sketch your findings below:

# ZONE OF INHIBITION

NOTE: There are limitations to this test in the case of slow-growing organisms or anaerobic organisms regarding the standardized zone diameter which may be read for diagnostic purposes. If no change is observed, it may be beneficial to re-incubate for 12 more hours.

## California Mastitis Testing:

To perform the California Mastitis Test, you should have the following:
√ CMT 4-quarter testing paddle **(Figure 15-3)**
√ CMT reagent
√ Warm water
√ Disposable paper towels
√ Gloves

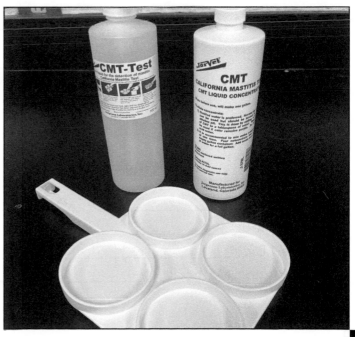

Figure 15-3: California Mastitis Test (CMT) paddle. Each paddle has four shallow cups used to collect milk from each of the udder quadrants. Place about 1 teaspoon of milk in each cup. After milk collection add an equal part of CMT solution to each cup. Rotate the paddle which mixes the milk and solution. Pay attention to time as a reaction, manifested by a thickening or presence of "gel", generally occurs within 10 to 20 seconds.

Restrain the animal in such a way as to gain ease of access to the udder and teats, it is suggested that there be a dedicated restrainer at the head of the animal to maintain safe control during collection. Gently wipe the teat/udder area in a downward motion with a warm water soaked towel. Do not "scrub" the area.

Holding the paddle under the animal so that the handle points to the tail and the teats are aligned with the collection areas, express a small amount of milk (approximately .5 to 1 teaspoon) from each udder into the corresponding cup on the paddle. Once collection is completed, add an equal amount of CMT reagent to the cup and begin to rotate it mixing the milk and reagent. Pay close attention to the timing and after rotating the sample for ten seconds look for a reaction. A positive reaction is manifested by a thickening or presence of "gel" within the mixture. Because this reaction occurs rapidly, you should expect to see positive results within 10 to 20 seconds of swirling. Based on the timing and observation, it is possible to assign a score of severity of mastitis for each animal tested **(Table 15-1)**.

### TABLE 15-1
### Severity Of Mastitis

| OBSERVATION | WHAT IT MEANS | SCORE |
|---|---|---|
| No thickening or gel present. | Animal has 100,000 cells or less per ml of milk. Deemed negative. | N = negative |
| Slight thickening observed for approximately 10 seconds. | Early traces of mastitis, animal has 100,000 to 300,000 cells per ml of milk. Deemed to be a "trace". | T = trace |
| Distinct thickening lasting over 10 seconds, no gel formation. | Animal has 300,000 to 900,000 cells per ml of milk. | 1 |
| Immediate and distinct thickening as well as formation of gelatinous matter. | Animal has high levels of cells per ml of milk of approximately 2,700,000. | 2 |
| Formation of gel, thick enough to stick to paddle and "peak" like a meringue. | Animal has approximately 8,100,000 cells per ml of milk or more. This is a definite unhealthy cell count. | 3 |

# LAB REPORT
# ANALYSIS OF MILK

**Milk Collection**

Animal Identification:_____

Date/Time:_____

Teat Sampled:_____

Collected By:_____

Transportation Method:_____

1. Microscopic Examination: Please draw and identify to the best of your ability, the microorganisms which are viewed. Answer the following to indicate presence:

Bacilli (rods): _____

Cocci (spherical): _____

Spirillum (spirals): _____

2. Cell Enumeration (over the course of 5 fields, show your work)

Field I:_____

Field II:_____

Field III:_____

Field IV:_____

Field V:_____

Total/f =_____ APF (average per field)

APF (microscopic factor) = microbial count per ml.

APF:_____

3. Standard Plate Count: (CFU's):

Plate #1: _____ CFU

Plate #2:_____ CFU

Plate #3:_____ CFU

Plate #4:_____ CFU

Plate #5:_____ CFU

Discuss the results of the CFU (colony forming units) above. What is the relationship between the dilution factors and the numbers of colony forming units for the 5 plates inoculated?

4. Within the circle, indicate the disk contents as well as sketching any zones of inhibition noted.

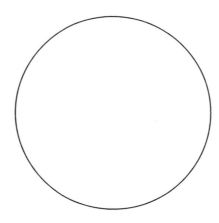

Within the chart below, fill in the information based on your observation.

| DISK | Antibiotic | Zone Measured (mm) |
|------|------------|--------------------|
| A    |            |                    |
| B    |            |                    |
| C    |            |                    |
| D    |            |                    |

5. California Mastitis Test: Please complete the following:

Animal Species: _____

Animal Identification:_____

Teat Sampled: _____

Collection Date/Time: _____

Results:_____

Discuss your interpretation of California Mastitis Test results. Include any applicable medical history of the animal from which the sample was collected.

_____
_____
_____
_____
_____
_____
_____
_____

# REFERENCES

1. Hendrix, C., & Sirois, M. (2007). Laboratory Procedures for Veterinary Technicians. St. Louis: Mosby-Elsevier.

2. Holtgrew-Bohling, K. (2012). Large Animal Clinical Procedures for Veterinary Technicians. St. Louis, MO: Elsevier-Mosby.

3. Mellenberger, R. (2021, May 1). California Mastitis Test (CMT) An Invaluable Tool for Managing Mastistis. Retrieved as of 9-6-2021 from: https://immucell.com/wp-content/uploads/2017/05/An-Invaluable-Tool.pdf

4. Marshall RT. Dairy Foods: Producing the Best (2021, May 1). https://extension.purdue.edu/4h/Documents/dairy-foods-booklet.pdf

5. NA. (2021, May 1). Fluid Milk Consumption in the United States. Retrieved on 9-6-2021 from: https://www.statista.com/statistics/184240/us-per-capita-consumption-of-fluid-milk-products/

6. USDA. (2021, May 1). Milk Production reports. Retrieved from USDA website on 9-6-2021: https://usda.library.cornell.edu/concern/publications/h989r321c

# CHAPTER 16

## INTRODUCTION TO CYTOLOGY

# OBJECTIVES

This lab introduces the student to basic collection and staining techniques that are commonly performed within clinical veterinary practice. The lab addresses the following Veterinary Technician Student Essential and Recommended Skills as set forth by the AVMA-CVTEA in Appendix 1 – Section 6: Laboratory Procedures:

√ Assist in collection, preparation and evaluation of transudates, exudates and cytological specimens

√ Assist in collection, preparation and evaluation of ear cytology

√ Assist in collection, preparation and evaluation of canine vaginal smears

# KEY TERMS

Adenocarcinoma

Anestrus

Anisokaryosis

Benign Neoplasm

Biopsy

Bronchial Wash

Centesis

Cornified Squamous Epithelial Cells

Cystocentesis

Diestrus

Estrus

Exudate

Fine Needle Aspirate

Granulomatous Inflammation

Imprint

Isotonic Fluid

Malignant Neoplasia

Neoplasia

Non-Cornified Squamous Epithelial Cells

Pleomorphic

Proestrus

Pyogranulomatous Inflammation

Romanowski Stains

Sarcoma

Scraping

Squash Prep

Starfish Smear

Suppurative Inflammation

Swab

Trans-Tracheal Wash

Transudate

Tzanch Technique

# INTRODUCTION

Cytology is the study of cellular elements of tissue, organs and other areas of the body. We refer to the study of cells that have been shed from a body structure as "exfoliative cytology" (**Figure 16-1**). This may include the examination of cells in fluid such as cerebrospinal, peritoneal, pleural, and ocular fluid (i.e. tears and aqueous or vitreous humor). The following are some common cytological collection and preservation methods that veterinary technicians frequently encounter within the scope of clinical practice:

√ Vaginal swabbing

√ Ear swabbing

√ Nasal swabbing

# DISCUSSION

The collection of cytologic specimens regardless of the origin must be done with attention to detail regarding aseptic technique because of the possibility of contamination. These specimens will be utilized for diagnostic purposes and therefore could become problematic if performed improperly. Asepsis should be practiced before, during and after all collections to minimize contamination.

It is equally important to recognize the most appropriate manner in which to carry out a cytologic collection. The following are some of the more common methods used in clinical practice. The technician should not only be familiar with the clinical technique but also be able to ascertain with a degree of certainty, which method is best suited for individual circumstances. While the practicing veterinarian will ultimately decide on the procedure, it behooves the well-trained technician to be familiar with the methodologies and the supplies required in order to facilitate a well-organized clinical experience.

Students completing this lab will have the chance to become proficient within the following Veterinary Technician Student Essential and Recommended Skills as set forth by the AVMA-CVTEA in Appendix 1 – Section 6: Laboratory Procedures:

√ Assist in collection, preparation and evaluation of transudates, exudates and cytological specimens.

√ Assist in collection, preparation and evaluation of ear cytology.

√ Assist in collection, preparation and evaluation of canine vaginal smears.

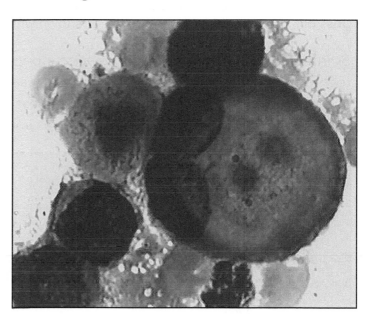

Figure 16-1: Exfoliative cytology is the study of cells shed by the body. Here are abnormal transitional cells, from a transitional cell carcinoma, in the urine of a dog.

# Techniques of Cytological Collection
## Swabs:
Used for sampling, which is not conducive to scraping, aspirating or imprints, this includes sampling of areas such as the vagina, ear and nose **(Figure 16-2)**. It is important to consider the comfort of the animal when "swabbing" by using a moistened swab. An appropriate moistening agent is sterile isotonic saline (0.9%) which will aid in comfortable collection and reduce damage to cells. Swabbing should be done gently, and you should never insert a swab into an orifice that is not plainly visualized. Cellular components can be retrieved by passing the swab over the involved area. Next gently roll the swab over a clean microscope slide without rubbing which will damage cells by friction and make them impossible to identify. If the swab is to be shipped to an outside lab, it should be preserved using a Culturette® for preservation and protection during transport.

## Scrapings:
The process of scraping is used on tissues which require collection of many cells or organisms that are not normally found on the tissue surface. When the scraping technique is utilized in superficial tissue (i.e. epidermis), the results are often indicative of a secondary bacterial infection

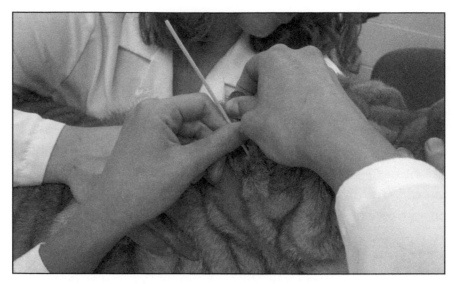

Figure 16-2: Swabs are best used in areas where scraping, aspirating or direct impression smears are not possible such as within the ear canal as shown with this dog.

or inflammatory response that may occur because of parasites. For this reason, the sampling technique is best restricted to suspected cases of problems such as derrmal parasites and inflammation induced dysplasia of tissue. The most common use of this technique is in the identification of dermal parasites such as *Demodex* and *Sarcoptes* mites **(Figure 16-3)**.

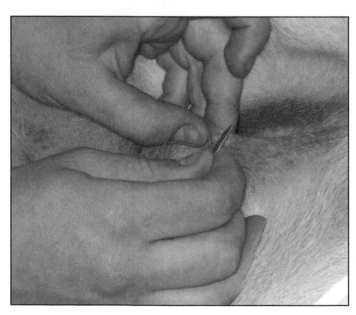

Figure 16-3: Skin scraping techniques are best accomplished with a sterile blade and used to gently scrape affected skin from bleeding tissue. As some parasites are found within, and not just on top of, the skin the scrape technique should break through the outer layer of the skin and induce a small amount of bleeding. If done properly, this should cause minimal pain to the animal.

## Imprints:
There are a few different ways in which an imprint of cytologic specimens can be created. The simplest procedure is to make multiple impression slides of a lesion and its visible exudate. The most time consuming procedure is to make a series of imprints of an external lesion characterized by scabbing, known as the Tzanch Technique. The advantage of the Tzanch Technique is the lack of sedation needed for patients and the ease of collection. The disadvantage is the likelihood of contamination of the sample due to extraneous bacterial and cellular debris which will also be collected during the procedure **(Figure 16-4)**.

There are other techniques for cytological collection that are a bit more invasive and some of them require sedation or mild tranquilization. These are best left to the expertise of the practicing veterinarian with an able technician to assist. **Table 16-1** provides a list of supplies which will be needed for specific types of sampling:

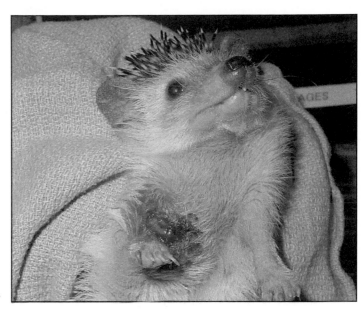

Figure 16-4: Direct impression smears are best for easily accessible skin wounds such as this ulcerative mammary lesion in a hedgehog. The slide is placed over and gently pressed on the skin lesion to create an 'impression smear'. While easy to perform, impression smears often pick up surface contamination that must be considered when interpreting the cytologic findings.

| TABLE 16-1 Cytology Techniques And Supplies | |
|---|---|
| **TECHNIQUE** | **SUPPLIES** |
| Swabs | Sterile cotton or rayon swabs<br>0.9% saline (isotonic)<br>Culturette (for shipping)<br>Microscopic slides<br>Quik-Dip or other Romanowski stains<br>Microscope |
| Scrapings | Scalpel blade<br>Microscope slides<br>Quik-Dip or other Romanowski stains<br>Microscope |
| Imprints | Microscope slides<br>Quik-Dip or other Romanowski stains<br>Microscope |
| Fine Needle Biopsy | 21 to 25 gauge needle (**Figure 16-5**)<br>3 to 20 mL syringe<br>Microscope slides<br>Quik-Dip or other Romanowski stains<br>Microscope |
| Punch Biopsy | Punch biopsy tool (**Figure 16-6**)<br>Forceps<br>Wooden tongue depressor<br>Formalin in jar (preservative) |

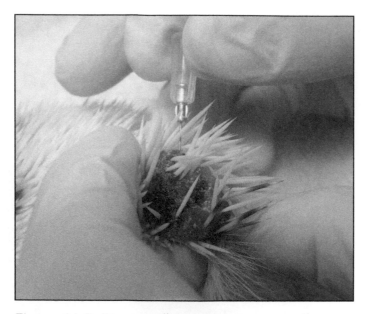

**Figure 16-5:** Fine needle aspirate is an excellent means of collecting cells from solid masses. Once the sample is collected, a syringe is attached to the needle and the contents are forcibly expelled onto a slide. This hedgehog skin mass is being aspirated with a 25g needle.

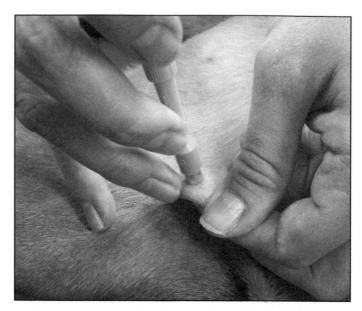

**Figure 16-6:** Circular punch biopsy tools are commonly used to collect small skin biopsy samples. While the image shows the procedure on normal dog skin and is for demonstration purposes only, skin biopsies should be performed under sterile conditions and with local or general anesthesia.

# LABORATORY SESSION

## INTRODUCTION

Cytology collection is often used when there is a need to examine cellular levels of inflammation or infection. It is essential to understand the correct methodology involved in collection, handling and preservation of specimens before sampling is attempted.

## MATERIALS AND SUPPLIES

Cotton swabs

Dog muzzle

Hair dryer

Microscope

Microscope slide

Quik-Dip stain

Saline

Vaginal speculum

## Lab Assignment

This lab is designed to acquaint the student with the various types of cytologic collection and examination methods used in clinical veterinary medicine on a regular basis. Students should be organized in groups of 2 and retrieve a female dog for collection purposes. Remember to log all activities and observed results of the cytologic testing in the patient records. The collection of animal tissues should take place in a clinical/treatment area while the staining and examination of slides will be performed in a clinical laboratory setting to avoid contamination of the samples.

## Ear Cytology (E):

Utilizing a clean swab, collect exudate from the outer ear and roll it onto a microscope slide. Use a hair dryer on the low setting to melt any wax that is observed in the sample. Once the slide is dry, it should be labeled (E) and set aside for staining in the pathology lab using Quik- Dip® or other Romanowski stain **(Figures 16-7 & 16-8)**.

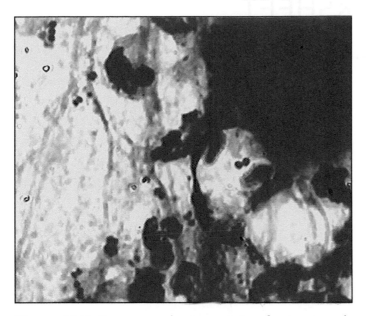

Figure 16-7: Romanowsky type stain of an ear swab from a dog. The slide has neutrophils and paired cocci consistent with bacterial otitis externa.

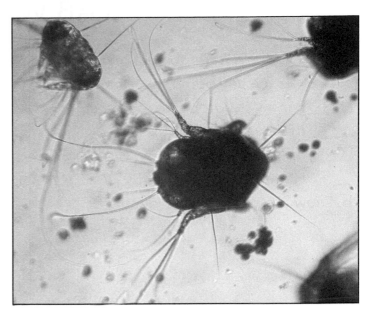

Figure 16-8: Ear mites (*Otodectes sp*) are common findings in cats, dogs, ferrets and other animals. These mites are best found in dark ear exudate that is collected via a swab and then transferred to a glass slide.

## Vaginal Cytology (V):

Utilizing a clean swab and speculum, prepare the dog for vaginal collection by standing the dog up and inserting the warmed speculum into the vaginal opening. Once a clear view is established, pass the moistened swab into the vaginal vault and gently swab the area. Withdraw the swab and roll it over a microscope slide, do not rub as cells will be destroyed. Label the slide (V) and air dry, setting it aside for staining with Quik-Dip® or other Romanowski stain.

## Nasal Cytology (N):

Gently but firmly restrain the dog, allowing it to face the collector. Advance a moistened swab gently into the nares while rotating the swab before withdrawing it (animal may sneeze). Roll the swab onto a slide and air dry the slide, label it (N) and set it aside for staining with Quik-Dip® or other Romanowski stain.

## Staining:

Utilizing previously learned techniques; stain the slide using the Quik-Dip® three-step system. Once the slide is blotted dry, view it under a microscope and complete the worksheet.

# INTRODUCTION TO CYTOLOGY
# LAB WORKSHEET

1. Ear Cytology: Refer to your textbook and answer the following:

a. Do you see any of the following:

_____ Ear mites (*Otodectes* species)

_____ *Malassezia* organisms

_____ Epithelial cells

_____ Hematological cells (RBC, WBC)

b. Draw any components identified.

2. Vaginal Cytology: Refer to your textbook and answer the following:

a. Can you identify what stage of estrus the animal is in, justify your answer.

b. Draw any cellular components which you have identified.

c. What other things have you identified on this slide, if any?

3. Nasal Cytology: Refer to your textbook and answer the following:

a. Upon examination of the slide, do you see any neutrophils?

b. What types of bacteria are present?

c. Draw any organisms or objects that you can identify.

## REFERENCES

1. Freeman, K. (2007). Veterinary Cytology of the Dog, Cat, Horse and Cow. London: Manson Publishing.
2. Hendrix, C., & Sirois, M. (2007). Laboratory Procedures for Veterinary Technicians. St. Louis: Mosby-Elsevier.
3. Meyer, D. (2004). Veterinary Laboratory Medicine - Interpretation and Diagnosis, 3rd Ed. St. Louis: Saunders.
4. Valenciano, A. (2014). Cowell and Tyler's Diagnostic Cytology and Hematology of the Dog and Cat. St.Louis: Elsevier.

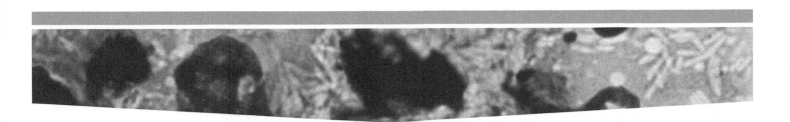

# CHAPTER 17

## CYTOLOGY: THE ART OF FINE NEEDLE ASPIRATION

# OBJECTIVE

This lab covers the "art" of fine needle aspiration. This procedure may be performed on peripheral lymph nodes, organs such as the liver, masses or other suspicious areas. The purpose is to sample the mass for a collection of cells from within the lesion or suspicious tissue in order for the clinician to diagnose and subsequently treat the animal appropriately.

This lab addresses the following Veterinary Technology Student Essential and Recommended Skills List as set forth by the AVMA-CVTEA in Appendix I, Section 6 – Laboratory Procedures Specimen Analysis to include:

Perform cytological evaluation
√ Perform fine needle aspirate and impression smear preparation (differentiate benign from malignant)

## KEY TERMS

Benign
Cytology

Fine Needle Aspirate
Fine Needle Biopsy

Malignant
Negative Pressure

# CYTOLOGY-FINE NEEDLE ASPIRATE LAB 17

# INTRODUCTION

Cytological examinations may be carried out either by fine needle biopsy (FNB) or fine needle aspirate (FNA) and may be performed on any organ or tissue. While an aspirate may be performed by a licensed veterinary technician, the needle biopsy is typically performed by a licensed veterinarian and in many cases is considered a surgical technique. The fine needle biopsy is used to collect a sample and requires a large bore needle while the sample collected for an aspirate requires a smaller needle for histological preparation. In addition to the collection technique, one must also understand the preservation method for samples collected via either technique for observation, and diagnostics. Students should understand various staining techniques as they relate to cytology.

## Discussion

According to the AVMA-CVTEA guidelines entitled Veterinary Technology Student Essential and Recommended Skills List, Section 6: Laboratory Procedures – the veterinary technician should be able to perform the following tests:

√ Perform fine needle aspirate and impression smear preparation (differentiate benign from malignant)

In order to fulfill this challenge, students should be capable of performing this technique, to assist others who may be performing needle aspirates, and be able to create a smear appropriate for staining.

# Fine Needle Aspirate:

This is generally accomplished by two people; a restrainer and a collector. The animal must be firmly but humanely restrained so that access is granted to the person carrying out the collection. For optimal collection and comfort, a 22 to 25 gauge needle and a 3 to 20 mL syringe should be used.

The mass should be stabilized with one hand while the needle is inserted into the center of the mass with the other hand. Immediately withdraw the plunger approximately 3/4 of the way into the syringe barrel causing negative pressure while moving the needle in a back and forth motion within the mass. Be careful not to pierce the opposite side of the mass or exit the mass while performing this maneuver to avoid possible aspiration of contamination into the barrel of the syringe and rendering the aspirate sample useless. Also, do not allow the needle to slip out of the mass into surrounding tissues during aspiration to avoid possible contamination.

Once satisfied with the collection, cease aspiration, and withdraw the needle from the mass (taking care not to depress the plunger). Remove the needle from the syringe and fill the syringe with air before replacing the needle. With the needle poised over a clean microscope slide, gently but forcefully expel air through the syringe/needle forcing the contents onto the slide **(Figure 17-1)**. This should be repeated several times in order to create several slides of stainable quality. If the slides are being shipped to an outside laboratory, check with the facility for their requirements regarding the staining of prepared slides. While you may or may not stain the specimen before mailing, many labs prefer to stain slides on site and will advise you of the best course of action.

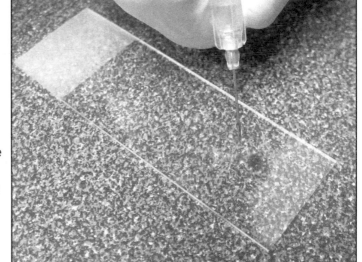

Figure 17-1: After performing the needle aspirate make the cytology slide. Unless a lot of fluid was collected during the aspirate, most of the cellular material will be in the needle hub and needle itself. Detach the needle from the syringe. Fill the syringe with air before reattaching needle and then gently but forcibly expel the cellular contents onto a clean glass slide.

An alternative method involves the use of a needle without the syringe for the collection. A 25-gauge needle is inserted into the mass and rapidly advanced and withdrawn ten to twenty times while keeping the needle entirely within the mass and without the use of suction from a syringe. The collected cells are packed into the bore of the needle where they are stored until the needle is withdrawn. Using a syringe, the contents of the needle can be expelled onto the slide for staining as described above. Diagnostically it is always a good idea to collect cells from at least two locations within the mass to increase the odds of collecting cells that are characteristic of the mass.

Once placed on the slide, the sample must be prepared for staining. This may be done by one of the squash preparations or "starfish" preparation method. For a refresher on the technique of making a blood smear which can be used for liquid or extremely moist samples, refer to Chapter 5.

In preparation for cytological analysis of the collected sample(s), a squash prep is performed **(Figure 17-2)**. The two types of 'squash preps' are known as a 'horizontal pull apart' and a 'vertical pull apart'. Both involve 'squashing' the expelled material between two slides. A horizontal pull apart is best for tough or thick samples (fibrous tumors) but can result in more ruptured cells. A vertical pull apart is best for delicate tissue (lymph nodes) but can result in more cell clumping. If unsure, first perform a vertical pull apart. If the cells are still too thick, then a horizontal pull apart can be performed on the same sample(s).

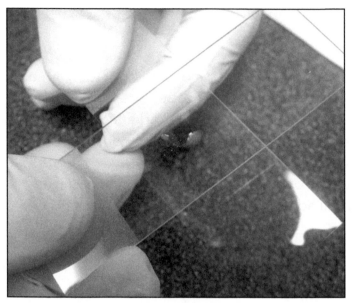

Figure 17-2: Once the cytologic specimen has been expelled on to the slide perform a 'sqaush prep' with another clean slide. First squash the two slides together. Next perform either a horizontal or vertical pull apart. A vertical pull apart involves directly pulling the slides apart from each other without any sliding motion. These are best for delicate cells such as with lymph node aspirates. A horizontal pull apart involves sliding the two slides apart from each other creating a smear of material. These are best with tough solid tissues because the shearing is needed to isolate individual cells.

A vertical pull apart is performed as follows: the expelled sample is placed in the center of the slide. A second slide (perpendicular) is firmly pressed down on the sample. The second slide is then pulled vertically off the first. This should create similar squash marks on both slides. Both slides can be air dried for staining **(Figures 17-3 and 17-4)**.

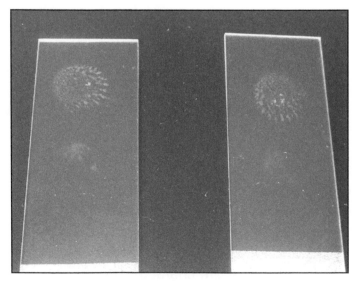

Figure 17-3: Vertical pull apart showing similar 'squash' marks on both slides.

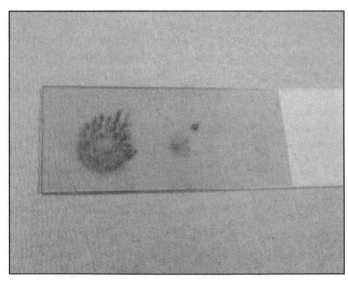

Figure 17-4: Vertical pull apart slide stained with Dip-Quick stain showing the 'squash' mark.

A horizontal pull apart is performed as follows: The expelled sample is placed in the center of a slide before placing another slide on top of the first slide (perpendicular) and firmly pressing down while drawing the top slide in a downward motion (advancing to the end of the slide). If done correctly, the sample will spread out and form a flame pattern similar to that seen with blood smear preparations. Both slides can be air dried for staining **(Figure 17-5)**.

The "starfish prep" is sometimes used for creating a stainable smear by using the point of the collection needle. By dragging the needle through the discharged sample on the slide in several directions, it is possible to create a starfish pattern of multiple points or projections. The slide is then air dried and stained.

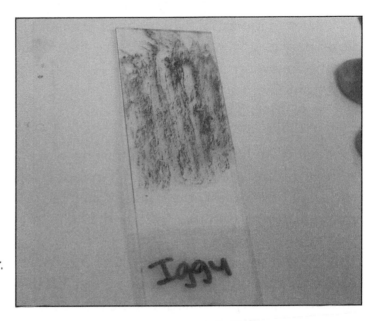

Figure 17-5: Stained slide after a horizontal pull apart. The slide is being dried on bibulous (or blotting) paper. Note the spread of cellular debris across the length of the slide.

## Staining:

There are different types of laboratory stains which may be effectively used. The most popular cytological stains are the Romanowski stains which include Wright's Stain, Giemsa Stain and the Diff-Quick (or Quik Dip® [Mercedes Medical]) staining system). The Papanicolaou Stain (commonly known as "pap stain") is also very popular. However, Romanowski stains are the most commonly used in veterinary practice. To achieve the best results, follow the instructions included with the stain. It is not advisable to mix various stains or make substitutions as this will affect the results.

Some helpful hints regarding the use of stains for best results:
√ Use only clean slides.
√ Use fresh stains for best results.
√ Used stains may be strained to remove debris and "freshen".
√ Slides must be completely dry before staining.
√ Do not stack slides or store so that the slides touch as this may mar the surface of the slide.
√ Store slides (completely dry) standing on end in a stain box.
√ Mail slides in a slide box (if possible) where they are standing and not touching. Avoid flat slide mailers, if at all possible, to avoid breaking or damaging the slide during mailing or transport.

# LABORATORY SESSION
# FINE NEEDLE ASPIRATION CYTOLOGY

## INTRODUCTION

The preparation of a cytological specimen in order to interpret a sample at the cellular level is of utmost importance. Correct, aseptic collection is the first step towards a diagnostic quality slide. Collect a sample following the instructions on the laboratory report and place it on a clean microscope slide. Repeat the process until you have at least 2 slides for staining purposes. Allow the slides to air dry completely before staining per your instructor's direction. You may expect to utilize at least one (possibly two) types of Romanowski stains (Papanicolaou Stains are not often used in veterinary clinical medicine). Follow the manufacturers' instructions or consult Lab # 4 for directions for the following:

√ Wright-Giemsa Stain
√ Quik-Dip (Diff-Quick) Stain

Once you are familiar with the staining procedures, you may begin to stain your slides for examination and complete the following lab report for submission to your instructor. An ideally prepared slide will have readily distinguishable intact and evenly stained cells in evidence when examined microscopically **(Figures 17-6 and 17-7)**.

HINT: Refer to your textbook or other reference books for identification of stained cells. Among references that may be helpful are the following:

√ Cowell and Tyler's Diagnostic Cytology of the Dog and Cat, 5th Ed.
√ Veterinary Cytology – Dog, Cat Horse and Cow

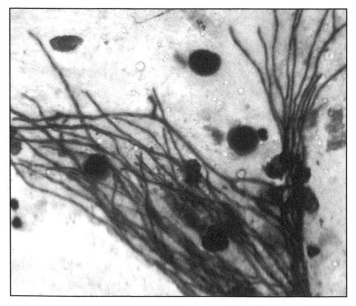

**Figure 17-6:** Diff-Quick® (Romanowsky type) stain of fungal elements. Note the even staining of the cellular components.

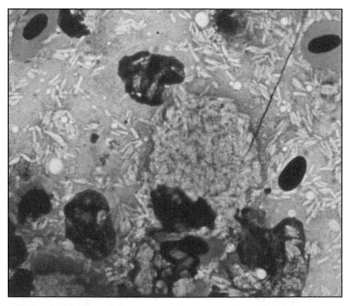

**Figure 17-7:** Diff-Quick® (Romanowsky type) stain of tuberculosis type bacteria. Note the even staining of the cells. These types of bacteria do not stain with Romanowsky type stains leaving 'ghosts' of the rods.

# FINE NEEDLE ASPIRATE

## CYTOLOGY WORKSHEET

1. Collect a sample from a mass aseptically, referring to directions in the aforementioned instructions within this chapter.

2. Transfer the sample to 2 clean microscope slides and using the starfish or squash (vertical and horizontal) prep methods, spread the sample thinly on the slide and allow it to air dry.

3. Utilizing the Diff-Quik (Quik-Dip) method, stain one slide and set it aside to dry after blotting (do not rub).

4. Utilizing the Wright-Giemsa method, stain the second slide and set it aside to dry after blotting (do not rub).

5. Within the circles below, draw the cells that you observe and attempt to identify them using your reference resources. Also describe their appearance.

Quik-Dip (Diff-Quick):

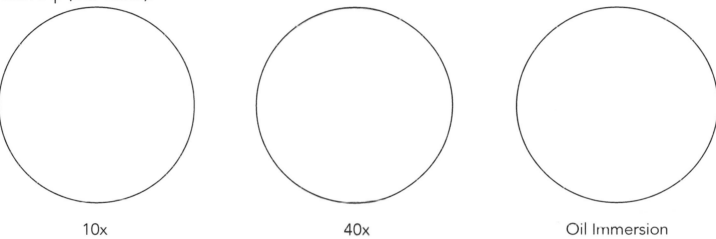

|          |          |               |
|:--------:|:--------:|:-------------:|
| 10x      | 40x      | Oil Immersion |

Wright-Giemsa Staining:

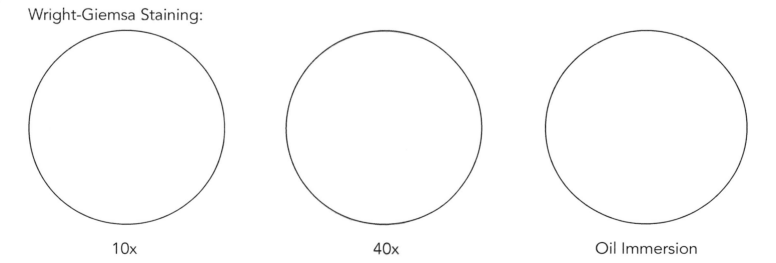

|          |          |               |
|:--------:|:--------:|:-------------:|
| 10x      | 40x      | Oil Immersion |

1. Answer the following questions regarding cytology and fine needle aspiration.

    a. Which staining method yielded the best results, why?_____

_____

_____

    b. Utilizing your textbook and other references, can you identify the types of cells seen on Slide #1 and Slide # 2?_____

_____

_____

    c. Upon inspection of each slide, what pathological evidence, if any, is there on each slide that you can identify?_____

_____

_____

    d. Upon inspection of each slide, do you find evidence of human error in smear content or preparation (i.e. traumatized cells, fragmented nuclei, ruptured or crenated cells, and scratches)?

_____

_____

_____

    e. Examine the two staining solutions; do they appear fresh and uncontaminated? How would you expect an overused, contaminated stain to look?_____

_____

_____

    f. Using gauze draped over a glass beaker, pick a stain and strain it. Examine the used gauze for contaminants and describe what you see? Why is this important?_____

_____

_____

# REFERENCES

1. Freeman, K. (2007). Veterinary Cytology of the Dog, Cat, Horse and Cow. London: Manson Publishing.
2. Hendrix, C., & Sirois, M. (2007). Laboratory Procedures for Veterinary Technicians. St. Louis: Mosby-Elsevier.
3. Valenciano, A. (2020). Cowell and Tyler's Diagnostic Cytology and Hematology of the Dog and Cat 5th Ed. St. Louis: Elsevier.

City/State/Zip_____

Phone (        ) _____ Date Mailed _____

Doctor's Name_____

Owner's Name_____

DORSAL

VENTRAL

# CHAPTER 18

## NECROPSY: A TECHNICIAN'S ROLE

# OBJECTIVES

This lab introduces the student to the role of the veterinary technician during a necropsy; also known as the "animal autopsy". Although the veterinarian performs the actual necropsy, the veterinary technician performs important tasks which contribute to the diagnostic success of the procedure and the outcome (i.e. results). This is especially true when collecting and preserving specimens for later analysis.

Proper sample collection and storage and data recording should be emphasized. Sometimes definitive answers cannot be found on initial sample collection. With these inconclusive cases, saved tissues may need to be submitted for additional testing including electron microscopy, infectious disease identification, toxin diagnostics, etc. The field of veterinary forensic pathology is growing. Just like with human crime scene investigation, effective animal CSI is only as good as the information collected. Some cases turn into medical legal issues. Necropsies may go beyond simply identifying the cause of death and the procedure should be handled professionally. It should be noted that any samples that are to be tested utilzing PCR technologies, should not be preserved in formalin. These samples should be stored in plastic bag or jar and shipped with ice packs to keep cool using overnight shipping if at all possible.

This lab addresses the following Veterinary Technology Student Essential and Recommended Skills list as set forth by the AVMA – CVTEA in Appendix I, Section 6: Laboratory Procedures.
√ Perform necropsy procedures
- Perform postmortem examination/dissection on non-preserved animals
- Collect samples, store and ship according to lab protocols
- Explain how to handle rabies suspects and samples safely
- Handle disposal of dead animals appropriately

# KEY TERMS

Anomalies/Anomaly

Ante-Mortem

Autolysis

Decomposition

Degradation

In Situ

Ligature

Necropsy

Post-Mortem

Prosector

Umbilical Tape

# INTRODUCTION

A necropsy is the scientific and medical examination of an animal after death. This is most often completed to determine the cause of death and may be a procedure of not only diagnostic but legal relevance. For these reasons, it is important that all observations as well as samples collected are labeled and logged as to date, time, type of samples, animal ID, etc. Additionally, it is essential to maintain documentation of the owner's permission to carry out the post-mortem examination as well as to ascertain their wishes regarding body disposition (i.e. cremation, return for burial, other burial options). In cases with legal ramifications, it may be necessary to maintain a chain of custody for samples to ascertain lack of evidence tampering or storage of the body as "evidence" until the case has been decided.

# DISCUSSION

When a dead animal is presented for necropsy, the clock is literally ticking regarding sample degradation and its effects on clinical success. If there is an expected delay before the necropsy can be performed, it is important to adequately cool the body to slow decomposition of tisssues. While bodies should be cooled, they should never be frozen. Freezing may cause histological changes as well as changes in the appearance of anomalies which may interfere with the diagnostic quality and findings of the exam. In cases of suspected rabies (large or small animal), freezing of the brain prior to examination may negate the ability to test and report results of legal importance and should **never** be done. In small animal species, sealing the animal in a plastic bag with attached identification on the animal as well as the bag (before refrigeration) will decrease the rate of autolysis. Large animal species are not as easily preserved and often require "field" necropsies in order to complete sample collection and note findings quickly before decomposition occurs. It is especially important to quickly preserve ruminant samples due to the rapid decomposition caused by the microbe-filled rumen which continues to generate heat (for a period of time) after death which accelerates decomposition. This is especially significant with GI tissue samples or rumen fluid being collected.

Feathers, scales and fur can insulate against heat and cold. This means that a dry, refrigerated animal may continue to decompose **(Figure 18-1)**. For smaller animals, the body can be moistened with water to facilitate cooling prior to placing it in a bag and refrigerator and before the actual necropsy. This is especially useful if the necropsy cannot be performed immediately after death.

Once all of the forms are signed, and the body is collected and stored appropriately, preparation for the necropsy begins. While ideally the necropsy suite will be maintained in anticipation of a scheduled event, this is often not the case. Because the necropsy is often performed to establish the cause of an unexpected death, the necropsy will be unplanned and may be performed in an exam room, pasture or other currently unused space.

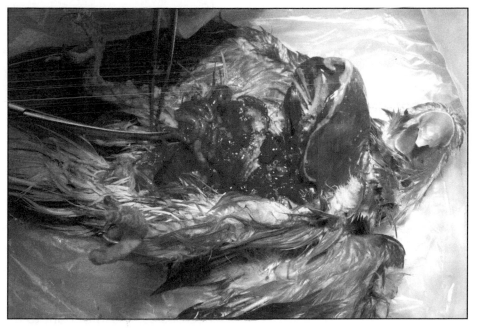

Figure 18-1: Feathers, scales and fur can insulate against cold slowing the cooling process when an animal is placed in the refrigerator prior to a necropsy. The outside of the body should be thoroughly wetted with water (as with this bird) prior to storing the animal in the refrigerator.

The veterinarian will want to review all records, logs and files pertaining to the case before starting and may wish to have a text of veterinary anatomy and physiology at the bench during the procedure. In most clinics the choice of where to perform a necropsy may be limited and the procedure may have to be conducted in the surgery suite, an exam room or outside (in the case of large animal species). For this reason, it is important to sanitize the necropsy area to provide a strictly aseptic environment both before and after the necropsy. It is not acceptable to use the surgery instruments for necropsy procedures – EVER. Necropsy tools and instruments should be kept separate from surgical instruments to avoid misuse; wherever possible, utilization of disposable supplies is advisable **(Figure 18-2)**. All disposables are to be treated as biohazards and discarded appropriately.

The ideal necropsy suite includes a designated area (room, corner of the building, etc.), ventilation hood, appropriate instruments, sample collection and storage devices (formalin jars, plastic bags, etc.) and personal safety equipment (gloves, masks, etc.) **(Figure 18-3)**. Of course, not every practice has a specifically designed necropsy suite. However, minimum equipment should include proper instruments, sample collection and storage devices and personal safety items. At a minimum, all personnel performing a necropsy or handling tissue should wear a mask and gloves. If infectious diseases are a concern, personal safety equipment may need to be upgraded to a gown, N95 respirator mask, protective eye wear and anything else deemed appropriate **(Figure 18-4)**.

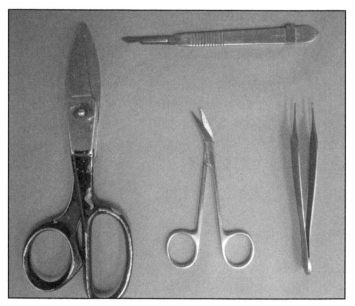

Figure 18-2: Necropsy instruments should be kept entirely separate from other instruments that might be used in surgery or clinical situations with live animals.

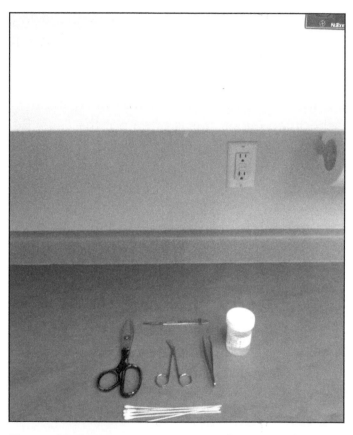

Figure 18-3: A necropsy suite or designated area is ideal for performing necropsies. Alternatively, a makeshift area, such as this covered countertop under a ventilation hood, may be used for necropsies. It is important to maintain cleanliness (sterility if possible) and take measures to prevent the spread of infectious materials to people, other patients and the necropsy patient itself.

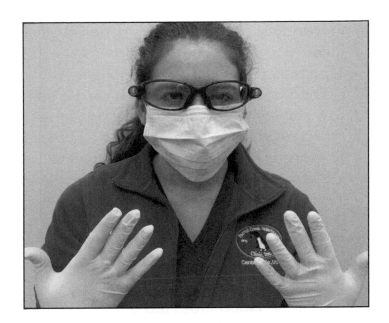

Figure 18-4: Personal protective equipment should be considered with all necropsies. The degree of protection depends on the condition of the animals and risk of infectious disease. At a minimum consider gloves, facemask and some type of eye protection.

# Instrumentation

It is important to have the correct tool for any job and a necropsy is no different. The size of the animal dictates the size and type of instrumentation required. Unlike a pristine "surgery", the necropsy is often physically taxing to the practitioner and in the case of large animals such as cows and horses requires brute strength to access areas of interest such as the thoracic or abdominal cavity. Because of the size of the animal (i.e. bone density and skin thickness) the instrumentation must either be a) delicate enough to avoid extraneous trauma to delicate tissue and fine bones or b) strong enough to provide enough force and energy to penetrate larger, denser tissues such as large animal bones and thickened cow hide. Never attempt to "make do" when assembling a necropsy pack; you will be setting up your practitioner for a frustrating journey into failure. It is recommended that a list be compiled of the instruments and supplies which a practitioner prefers and that it be posted for easy reference. These items should be labeled and maintained separately from other instruments and tools. They should never be used for surgical or treatment purposes.

## Large Animal Necropsy:

Many items used in a large animal necropsy are not actual surgical instruments but rather gardening tools which may be picked up at the local gardening or hardware store (such as pruning shears). Because of the size of the animal and the use of the occasional electrically powered saw, there is a real danger of aerosolized particulate contamination to those participating in the procedure. As with all animal necropsy or surgical procedures, precautions should be taken to avoid zoonotic spread of disease. For this reason, always have a supply of masks, gowns, gloves and face shields available and insist on their usage.

## Tools of the Trade: Large Animal Necropsy:

√ Knives of various blade types and sizes (similar to those used by professional butchers)
√ Whet-stone or sharpening/honing steel
√ Hatchett and/or hand-ax
√ Pruning shears
√ Scalpel handles and various sizes of blades
√ Sharps container

- √ Forceps (various sizes, toothed, non-toothed)
- √ Ruler
- √ Tape measure at least 10 feet long
- √ Cutting board (of a surface that can be sanitized with boiling water and/or autoclaved)
- √ Saw (variety to include hacksaw, Stryker saw, meat saw as well as extra blades)
- √ String or umbilical tape (for tying off bowels)
- √ Scissors (utility, Mayo and Metzenbaum)
- √ Collection buckets (preferably stainless steel)
- √ Tissues cassettes
- √ Buffered 10% formalin in sealable jars
- √ 50% formalin in sealable jars for complete organs **(Figure 18-5)**
- √ Ziploc bags, bottles, vials
- √ Red top blood tubes
- √ Purple top blood tubes (EDTA)
- √ Blue top tubes (Citrate)
- √ Needles (18 gauge 1.5", 16 gauge 1.5")
- √ Syringes (12 mL)
- √ Pens, Sharpie® markers
- √ Note paper and/or necropsy forms
- √ Paper towels
- √ Trash bags

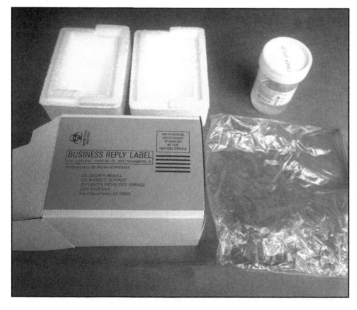

**Figure 18-5:** Formalin is the most commonly used fixative for storing tissues. Tissues should be no larger than 5 mm thick to ensure proper penetration and fixation with formalin. The tissue to formalin ratio should be 1:10 (1 part tissue, 10 parts formalin). Formaldehyde, the active ingredient in formalin, is highly toxic to all animals and is considered carcinogenic to humans. Formalin should be handled cautiously and be well packaged for shipping or transport to prevent leakage.

If the large animal necropsy is performed outside (as is often the case on farms) it is essential to thoroughly clean and sanitize the area after the procedure is completed. This often falls to the technician and the area should always be left in better shape than it was found. Some considerations include:

1. Wash and dry all buckets and other implements "borrowed" from the farm before returning them to the owner (to do this effectively keep a small bottle of dish detergent and paper towels handy).
2. Remove all trash and biological wastes (bag for disposal at farm trash cans).
3. If necropsy was done on a solid surface (concrete, etc.) wash it down with soapy water, rinse with 10% bleach solution and then thoroughly rinse with water.

4. If the necropsy was done on a grassy area, rinse the area thoroughly with water to remove any pools of blood or other bodily fluid to discourage flies, animals, etc. Pick up all organic and biological matter (organs, skin, etc.) and bag for disposal.

5. Pack up all instruments, supplies and samples checking the area twice to ensure that nothing is left behind.

6. All trash should be bagged with the bag tied shut and disposed of in farm garbage containers. Do not transport trash from the farm to avoid the spread of disease.

7. Rarely, the remaining carcass may need to be buried and/or burned. Either should only be performed with respect to local ordinances and laws or permission from the appropriate authorities.

## Small Animal Necropsy:

The main difference between a small animal necropsy and a large animal procedure is the size of the tools needed and the physical strength that is necessary. While the tools may be smaller, an electric bone saw is often needed which will require personal protective equipment (PPE's) such as protective eyewear and respiratory masks to prevent aerosolized contamination; insist on their usage.

## Tools of the Trade – Small Animal Necropsy:

√ Necropsy knives
√ Whet-stone/sharpening or honing steel
√ Scalpel handle and various sized blades
√ Sharps container
√ Forceps (toothed, non-toothed)
√ Ruler (metric system is most recognized scientifically) **(Figure 18-6)**
√ Tape Measure (4-foot length)
√ Small cutting board (can be sterilized)
√ String/umbilical tape
√ Scissors (utility, Mayo, Metzenbaum)
√ Collection buckets (stainless steel)
√ Tissue cassettes **(Figure 18-7)**
√ 10% formalin
√ Jars, sealable bags
√ Blood tubes (red to, purple top, [blue top – optional])
√ Plain glass tubes with stoppers (no preservative)
√ Needles of various gauges

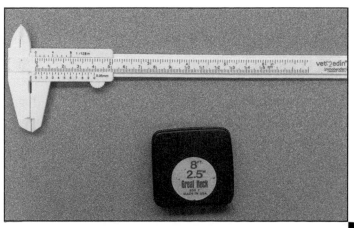

Figure 18-6: A metric system ruler and/or tape measure should always be available when performing necropsies. Organs, tissues and lesions may need to be measured and recorded (including with photographs) for basic medical records, studies and potentially even legal reasons.

√ Syringes (12 mL)
√ Pens, Sharpie® markers
√ Paper towels
√ Trash bags
√ Necropsy form/note paper

Small animal necropsies are often performed inside the surgery suites (especially if the animal died during surgery or while staying in the clinic), on an exam table or in a designated space or room. Every attempt should be made to ensure a sanitary and aseptic environment before, during and after the procedure. Because these rooms/tables are often utilized for medical treatment of living animals, it is imperative to maintain these areas in a disease-free, aseptic state at all times. Once a necropsy is completed and the carcass is disposed of, the entire area should be cleaned, disinfected and sanitized before other patients (dead or alive) are introduced to the area.

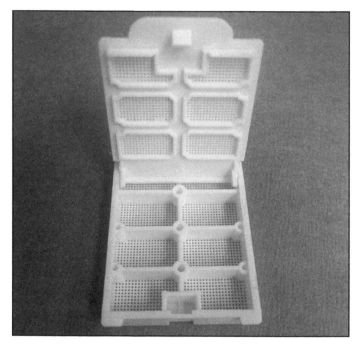

Figure 18-7: Tissue cassettes can be used to isolate small tissue samples. The small perforated cassettes are filled with tissue samples and then submerged in formalin jars.

# LABORATORY SESSION-NECROPSY

## INTRODUCTION

The technician is invaluable to the success of the necropsy. In addition to the clinical acumen of the veterinarian, the veterinary technician's ability to manage specimens assures that proper collection, preservation and shipping is carried out which in turn supports the accuracy of the test results. For this reason, technicians should familiarize themselves with the necropsy process and have a thorough understanding of the established protocols for receipt of samples by commercial laboratories. It is important to realize that protocols change from time to time (especially with regard to the preservation of samples) including such things as the institution of new requirements regarding packing and shipping of specimens.

## Discussion

This lab will focus on becoming proficient in the technician's role during the necropsy as dictated by AVMA-CVTEA guidelines which include:

√ Performing instructor-led postmortem examination on the non-preserved animal (as a group).

√ Collect samples, store and ship per lab instructions (as a group).

√ Handle disposal of the dead animal.

√ Explain/demonstrate safe handling of rabies suspect and associated samples.

## This lab Requires:

√ Appropriate sized containers for preservation of samples.

√ 1 freshly dead animal (large or small animal species).

√ 1 set of necropsy instruments for appropriately sized animal (large or small, see list within this lab).

√ Necropsy forms (available on internet as well as commercially).

√ Appropriate PPE's.

Because it falls under the purview of the veterinarian to complete the actual necropsy, this lab will not "instruct" on necropsy procedures but instead will serve as a learning environment for the student technician to practice and become proficient in their role within the procedure while observing the process. For further edification and education on the step-by-step process of necropsy, the technician student is referred to two excellent textbooks on the subject of necropsy procedures:

√ Large Animal Necropsy

• Veterinary Clinical Procedures in Large Animal Practice by J Rockett and S. Bosted (Delmar-Cengage Learning, ISBN13: 978-1-4018-5787-5).

√ Small Animal Necropsy

• McCurnin;s Textbook for Veterinary Technicians, 10th Edition, Bassert, J., Beal, A., Samples, OM (Elsevier, ISBN 9780323722001).

# LABORATORY EXERCISE NECROPSY

## INTRODUCTION

The veterinary technician plays an important as well as energetic role in the necropsy procedure. This includes pre-procedure set-up, procedural duties (sample receipt, preservation, packing, shipping, assist the veterinarian) and post-procedural clean-up and carcass disposal. As each case differs, instructors will modify the experience to provide sufficient learning experiences and the development of student skills in accordance with the AVMA-CVTEA listed essential skills.

## Discussion

This lab exercise is broken down into three parts as mentioned above. It is suggested that students be broken into groups of two with group members taking turns being the "action figure" (performing tasks and assisting) and the "recorder" (documentation). Your instructor will tell you which scenario is going to be implemented. Student groups will be assigned to either pre-procedural, procedure or post-procedural activities based on the scenario which is chosen. Although this limits the student's opportunity to perform all tasks, every effort should be made to encourage and allow everyone to observe all steps and procedures as they are happening. Remember, the AVMA-CVTEA recognizes within the Veterinary Technology Students Essential and Recommended Skills list that students will participate in necropsy proceedings as a group learning experience. Your instructor will make every effort to include as much individualized, active participation as possible regardless of the scenario chosen.

Once groups are established, the necropsy report should be an ongoing activity that is completed as the necropsy is occurring. Although a group may not actively complete each activity they should endeavor to report as accurately as possible (based on their observations) on each part of the lab report.

## SCENARIO I:

The course instructor will provide a fresh cadaver on which the necropsy will be performed by a veterinarian as well as indicate which necropsy form you should complete (both A and B are included at the end of the exercise).

## SCENARIO II:

Students will attend a necropsy performed by a veterinarian as scheduled by the instructor in a clinical setting (i.e. veterinary office/clinic, college of veterinary medicine, commercial laboratory). Students will complete the indicated necropsy form based on the experience.

## Pre-Procedural Activities

In preparation of the necropsy, during the "Pre-Procedure" the following should be considered:
1. Table should be raised/lowered to a comfortable level that accommodates the height of the veterinarian. Cover the table with an absorbent drape if no drainage trays are built into the table. If drainage trays are available, ensure there is a drain or bucket to catch fluids.

2. Small animals should be placed in dorsal recumbency with limbs loosely secured (similar to the ovariohysterectomy [AKA OHE] surgical position).

3. A large animal necropsy will often be performed outdoors in "field conditions". Make sure to have all supplies at hand as you may not be at the clinic but rather on a farm and cannot retrieve forgotten items.

4. Before the necropsy begins, be sure that you have the correct animal identification, signed consent forms and the owner's name confirmed for use in records and on specimen labels.

5. Before the necropsy begins, note the condition of the body including any noticeable injuries, photograph the animal in situ, if necessary, for documentation.

6. Before beginning the procedure, make sure you have all supplies close at hand and in a large enough quantity to avoid having to leave the necropsy to search for things. This is particularly important regarding towels, pens, markers, labels, bags, jars, tubes, etc.

7. Once the procedure begins, be prepared to take notes, receive specimens and assist the practitioner (sometimes simultaneously) according to your place on the team.

8. Have a digital camera charged and ready for any documentation which may be necessary. For legal purposes, ensure that the date/time stamps are properly set on the camera. For small specimens, include a metric system ruler in the picture for size reference.

9. If there may be a need for review of radiographs, have a light box on hand and hooked up to electricity or digital radiograph viewing station positioned so that the practitioner may refer to radiographs while working.

10. Have the animal's previous records, radiographs, lab results, etc. on the bench for quick referral.

11. Have a copy of an anatomy text on the bench for quick referral.

12. If Form A is utilized, complete and share it with your classmates.

13. Complete Form B describing findings of the necropsy.

## Procedural Period of Necropsy

The veterinary technician serves a variety of functions during the necropsy including receiving specimens, aiding in the necropsy when a second set of hands is necessary and charting the veterinarian's observations. Complete the following activities that are to be incorporated in Necropsy Form A.

A. Briefly sketch the position of the animal, the incisions made (indicate with dashed lines) and any pertinent landmarks.

B. In-Situ examination: Briefly describe the carcass as it appears before the dissection is begun.

**Table 18-1** describes the best way to handle, preserve and store specimens which may be collected during necropsy. The following should be noted regarding the receipt of samples:

## Blood:

Due to the time lapse between death and the necropsy, blood is often clotted or semi-clotted **(Figure 18-8)**. Blood should be stored in a red-top tube (no additive) and cooled until centrifugation can take place. If the blood is not clotted (newly deceased animal), attempt to draw enough blood to create a set of hematological samples for later analysis that includes a red top tube, purple top tube (EDTA) and a blue top tube (Citrate – optional for use in coagulation tests). It is also acceptable and recommended to make a set of at least 2 labeled blood smears at this time. These may be set aside to dry until time is available for staining them after the necropsy is completed. Be sure to package the smears in a slide mailer to avoid breakage and contamination (see chapters 4-9).

## TABLE 18-1
## Preservation Methods Of Necropsy Specimens

| SAMPLE | PRESERVATIVE | STORAGE VESSEL | POSSIBLE TESTS |
|---|---|---|---|
| Blood (clotted) | None | Red top tube | Biochemical profile, serum protein |
| Blood (unclotted) | EDTA | Purple top tube | CBC, platelets, smears |
| Blood (unclotted) | Heparin | Green top tube | CBC, electrolytes |
| Blood (unclotted) | Citrate | Blue top tube | Coagulation testing |
| Bones | 50% Formalin* | Glass jar, tightly sealed | Histological exam |
| Brain | 50% Formalin* | Glass jar, tightly sealed | Histological exam |
| Cytology specimen | None, complete smear & staining process | Prepared slide stored in slide box or mailer | Microscopic exam |
| Effusions (abdominal or thoracic) | EDTA | Purple top tube | Cell counts, physical observation, total protein, specific gravity |
| Fecal parasites | 70% Alcohol or 10% buffered formalin | Plastic or glass vial | Parasite identification |
| Feces | √ 10% formalin (if not to be examined for several hours) √ None (if to be examined immediately) | Plastic bag or vial. Always refrigerate if not examining immediately | Parasitology testing, blood, mucus |
| Otic cytology | None, complete smear and staining process | Swab, place in plastic bag until tested. Smear – slide box or mailer. | Cellular or bacterial identification, external parasite identification |
| Spinal cord (whole) | 50% formalin* | Glass jar, tightly sealed | Histological exam |
| Synovial joint fluid (store both) | EDTA | Purple top tube | Automated testing (cell counts) |
| Synovial joint fluid (store both) | None | Red top tube | Viscosity, mucin |

*50% formalin is made by combining 1 part 10% buffered formalin with 1 part commercial Formaldehyde.

## Urine:
If urine is aspirated from the bladder, make note of the amount and store it in a plain, labeled tube (glass or plastic) with no preservative and refrigerate immediately for later testing or shipment (see Chapter 3). Your veterinarian may wish to have the physical appearance of the urine recorded at the time of collection (i.e. color, clarity) (Figure 18-9). This should be done immediately.

## Tissue Samples:
Depending on the size of the tissue sample, it should be placed in a jar or tissue cassette with

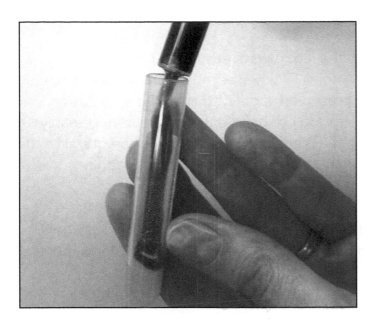

Figure 18-8: If possible collect blood from necropsy patients. Depending on the cause of death and condition of the carcass, blood may be clotted, semi-clotted or un-clotted. Mostly clotted blood can be saved in red top tubes, semi and un-clotted in purple top tubes and un-clotted in citrate tubes.

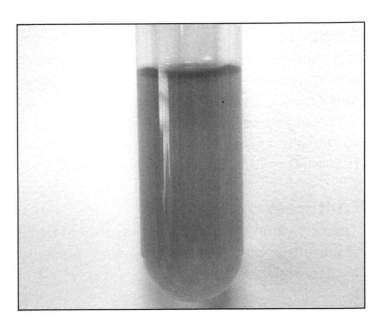

Figure 18-9: Collect urine for a post-mortem urinalysis. Also note the urine color, clarity, odor and any other pertinent physical characteristics as well as the volume collected.

10% formalin for preservation. It is imperative to label the sample with regard to animal identification, tissue type, date, and time of collection, immediately upon receipt because tissue is often unrecognizable as an organ once it is reduced to a 1 x 1 cm square. If the tissue is from a skin (tumor, lesion, etc.) note where exactly on the body the tissue was excised from in a rough drawing. This location is often diagnostically relevant **(Figure 18-10)**. Tissue samples should be no thicker than 1/5 of an inch (1/2 cm); both the tissue and the lesions sampled should be measured and recorded. Formalin can only penetrate 2 to 3 mm (from one side) so samples thicker than 0.5 cm (5 mm) may be improperly fixed and yield false histopathology results. Please note that any sample that is to be evaluated using PCR technology, should not be preserved in formalin or other preservatives. Instead, these samples should be fresh packaged and cooled for overnight transport.

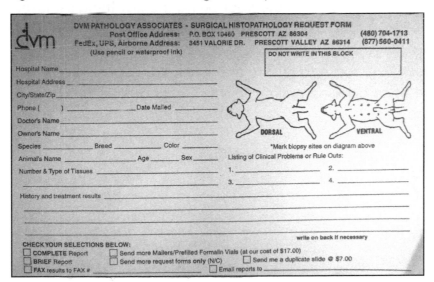

Figure 18-10: When collecting diagnostic samples from necropsy specimens, record the sample location, size and other pertinent physical characteristics. This information is also often requested on lab submission forms.

## Organs:

It is sometimes necessary to send the entire organ to the lab. Always ensure that you have a container large enough to sufficiently preserve the sample (10 times as much formalin as tissue) and prevent drying. If only part of an organ is being preserved, label it to avoid later confusion. With lung tissue, if collecting histopathological samples, do not handle the organ un-necessarily because this can cause diagnostically confusing artifacts. When submitting a large sample, slice the tissue (70 to 80% through) every 5 mm (0.5 cm, 1/5 inch) to allow proper formalin fixation.

## Cultures:

The collection of culture samples should be carefully and aseptically completed, preferably using Culturettes® that allow for collection, preservation and shipping in one device. Label the sample immediately.

# Post-Procedural Activities

At this point, the necropsy should be completed. Before moving the carcass, ensure that the veterinarian is finished and all samples that are needed have been collected. Do not forget to record the time of completion. The following must be completed as the post-procedure or "wrap-up".

1. Place the animal in a labeled cadaver bag and determine the final disposition instructions. All animals should be placed in either a cooler or freezer pending final disposal. If the owner has requested return of the animal, every effort should be made to clean the animal and present it in as natural an appearance as possible. If the animal is to be disposed of by the clinic, ensure that the owner has signed a consent form to that effect, consenting to final disposition by the clinic in whatever manner they deem appropriate.

2. Once the animal is moved, begin clean-up of the necropsy suite in the following manner:
   a. Remove all instruments for cleaning, disinfecting and lubrication before returning them to the necropsy pack.
   b. Clean the room starting high and ending low with disinfecting cleanser. Begin with the surgical lighting and work your way down with the floor being the last thing sanitized.
   c. All trash should be bagged and discarded outside; this includes all disposable products such as PPE's and draping.
   d. Make a final check of the room to ensure that it is ready for use. Eradicate any lingering odors with the discreet use of an odor neutralizing spray (i.e. Febreeze®).

# REVIEW QUESTIONS

Utilize available textbooks of instructor's choice to develop your answers to the following:

1. Is there a difference in the recumbency position of small animals as opposed to large animals for the purpose of a necropsy? Explain.

2. For what reasons do the prosector (attending veterinarian of the necropsy) typically remove the following organs for further "cutting board" dissection and examination?

    a. Heart:

    b. Kidney:

    c. Liver:

    d. Intestinal Tract:

    e. Reproductive Organs:

3. What types of zoonotic diseases might one expect to encounter in a small animal (species) necropsy? How should you protect yourself?

4. What types of zoonotic diseases might one expect to encounter in a large animal (species) necropsy? How should you protect yourself?

5. How should you handle a rabies suspect's carcass and samples safely, be specific and address handling as well as disposal?

6. How should dead animals (non-rabies suspects) be handled and disposed of to ensure safety?

7. How can the choice of euthanasia possibly impact the necropsy? Be specific.

8. Discuss humane euthanasia as it applies to the following:
   a. Large animal species (equine, bovine):

   b. Small ruminant species (i.e. caprine, ovine):

   c. Small animal species (i.e. canine, feline):

d. Lab animals (rodents, rabbits, guinea pigs):

9. Describe how to pack specimens for shipping via the U. S. Postal service as well as one other carrier such as UPS or Federal Express.

10. If a small or large animal is not being claimed for disposal, discuss acceptable methods of carcass disposal according to your state's regulations.

# NECROPSY REPORT FORM A

I. Pre-procedural Information:

A. General information:

B. Discuss the method of euthanasia and include justification for the method:_____
_____
_____

C. Based on your institutional/clinical setting, list tools of necropsy on hand for the procedure, include PPE's and collection vessels. This should be an all-inclusive list as set out in preparation for the necropsy._____
_____
_____
_____
_____

D. List reference texts placed bench-side for the veterinarian's use and provide a brief statement to indicate their value to the necropsy procedure._____
_____
_____
_____
_____

2. Procedural Information:

A. Briefly sketch the positioning of the animal and the incisions made.




B. Describe briefly the carcass as it appears before dissection (in situ):_____
_____
_____
_____

C. Describe any known medical history of the animal and prior, relevant lab reports._____
_____
_____
_____

D. Examine and note your observations of the external carcass and the appearance of the following:
Conformation:_____
Wounds or Lesions:_____
Hair Coat (condition of, evidence of ectoparasites):_____

E. Dissection:
a. Once incisions are made and the skin is reflected, name the superficial muscles which are encountered (HINT: A good anatomy text on the bench is helpful). You may want to sketch them also._____
_____
_____
_____

b. As the dissection continues, note any abnormalities that are pointed out by the veterinarian or prosector below:_____

_____

_____

_____

c. Note the condition of the organs of the thoracic cavity. What is the condition of the diaphragm? List each organ examined and its condition (NOTE: Have umbilical tape ready for ligation of the esophagus)._____

_____

_____

_____

d. Note the condition of the organs of the abdominal cavity. List each organ examined and its condition (NOTE: Have umbilical tape ready for ligation of the intestines). It may be helpful to have a cutting board available for dissection/examination of individual organs such as the spleen, heart, liver and kidneys._____

_____

_____

_____

e. The veterinarian (i.e. prosector) will determine how thorough the necropsy needs to be. Legal cases (i.e. abuse cases, wrongful death, etc.) will require a full and complete necropsy report while the owner of the pets (discovered dead for no reason) may only require investigation up to and including the immediate cause of death. From this point, please note all findings pointed out by the prosector for your report._____

_____

_____

_____

_____

_____

_____

F. Collection: List all samples which have been collected during the necropsy including how they are preserved. Refer to Table 18-1 for suggested preservation methods.

| SAMPLE | Size/Amount | Preservative | Storage Vessel | Refrigerate (yes/no) |
|---|---|---|---|---|
|  |  |  |  |  |
|  |  |  |  |  |
|  |  |  |  |  |
|  |  |  |  |  |
|  |  |  |  |  |
|  |  |  |  |  |
|  |  |  |  |  |
|  |  |  |  |  |
|  |  |  |  |  |
|  |  |  |  |  |
|  |  |  |  |  |
|  |  |  |  |  |
|  |  |  |  |  |
|  |  |  |  |  |

# NECROPSY REPORT FORM B

Instructions: This form requires more of a narrated report of what is found during the necropsy. Based on your observations, complete the following to the best of your ability; it is recommended that you may want to complete Form A also as a way to organize your thoughts before completing this report.

1. Signalment/History/Narration:_____
_____
_____
_____

2. Gross Findings:_____
_____
_____
_____

3. Laboratory Findings:_____
_____
_____

4. Diagnosis and Findings:_____

_____

_____

_____

5. Final Narrative:_____

_____

_____

_____

## REFERENCES

1. Bassert, J. (2014). McCurnin's Clinical TExtbook for Veterinary Technology, 8th Edition. St. Louis, MO: Elsevier.
2. Hendrix, C., & Sirois, M. (2007). Laboratory Procedures for Veterinary Technicians. St. Louis: Mosby-Elsevier.
3. Rockett, J. (2007). Veterinary Clinical Procedures in Large Animal Practice. Clifton Park, NY: Delmar-Cengage.
4. Studdert, V. G. (2012). Saunders Comprehensive Veterinary Dictionary, 4th Edition. New York, New York: Elsevier-Saunders.

# CHAPTER 19

## AVIAN, EXOTIC MAMMALS, REPTILES AND FISH

# OBJECTIVES

This lab exposes the student to the diverse world of avian and exotic animal (or non-traditional species) care. These animals may be seen in private practice, research, zoos, aviaries, private collections and in the field (wildlife). The veterinarian-technician team that works with these animals tends to be more specialized however general practitioners also may see avian and exotic species. Prior to working with non-traditional species, the student should have a basic understanding of husbandry, anatomy and handling to ensure proper evaluation and treatment of the species in question. This lab cannot adequately prepare the student for work with non-traditional species. However, resources will be offered to help interested students better understand care for these unique species.

Students interested in pursuing work with non-traditional species are encouraged to work alongside more experienced technicians and veterinarians through externships, internships, work-study programs and more.

In order to fully appreciate the veterinary technician's role in the collection, preservation and analysis of laboratory specimens this chapter is a bit more in-depth than previously covered topics which focused mainly on small and/or large animal species. Exotics including reptiles, fish, small mammals and avian species are often covered under the auspices of lab animal medicine at a minimal level. This chapter will be more inclusive regarding the role of the technician in the care of these animals including laboratory sampling and procedures.

This lab addresses the following Veterinary Technology Students Essential and Recommended Skills List as set forth by the AVMA-CVTEA in Appendix I, Section 9 – Avian, Exotic, Small Mammals and Fish Procedures:

√ Define and recognize animals that are 'non-traditional' species
√ Recognize basic concepts of handling, husbandry, behavior, collecting diagnostic samples, administering medications, anesthesia and analgesia and risks/legalities of owning non-traditional species
√ Perform basic collection of blood, urine, etc. on species as appropriate

# KEY TERMS

Capnography
Captive Wild Animal
Centers For Disease Control
Coelom
Domestic Animal
Electrocardiogram (ECG)
Feral Animal
Handling And Restraint
Husbandry

Intracoelomic Medications
Intraosseous Medications
Intravenous Medications
Invasive Animal
Local Anesthesia
Mentation
Non-Traditional Species
Ophthalmic Medications
Oral Medications

Pulse Oximetry
Regional Anesthesia
Renal-Portal System
Subcutaneous Medications
Systemic Anesthesia
Tame Animal
Topical Medications
Transdermal Medications
Wild Animal

# INTRODUCTION

'Non-traditional species' is the catch all term for animals not encountered in a 'traditional' practice setting. 'Traditional' animal medicine primarily centers on domestic animals that include cats, dogs, horses, cows, sheep, goats and pigs. This group of common animals is the focus of study in veterinary and veterinary technician schools in the developed world. While many animals such as chickens, turkeys, llamas and more have been domesticated for hundreds or even thousands of years, these animals are considered 'non-traditional'. Even mice and rats, which have been at the forefront of research and published studies and come from hundreds to thousands of generations raised in captivity, are considered 'non-traditional' species.

A non-traditional species can be domesticated, feral, wild, captive wild, invasive and/or tame. A domesticated animal is one that has been tamed and kept by humans for work, food or companionship and is notably different from their wild ancestors. For example, the ferret (*Mustela putorius furo*) was domesticated approximately 2,500 years ago from the European polecat (*Mustela putorius*) **(Figure 19-1)**. Ferrets are common pets in North America and Europe. A feral animal lives in the wild but descended from a domestic origin. For example, the common pet rabbit (*Oryctolagus cuniculus*) is a domestic descendant of the European rabbit (*Oryctolagus cuniculus*) and has colonized as feral populations in various parts of the world **(Figure 19-2)**. A wild animal lives without human intervention and has not been tamed. A black bear (*Ursus americanus*) roaming a national park is 'wild' whether it is friendly, aggressive or completely avoids people **(Figure 19-3)**. A Captive wild animal best describes the many exotic animal species kept as pets that are not domesticated and may or may not be tame. A pet blue and gold macaw (Ara ararauna) may have been raised in captivity, sociable and tame with people but has not truly been domesticated **(Figure 19-4)**. Invasive animals are those that freely live in a non-native habitat. While not always the case, invasive animals are often introduced by humans and can be domestic, feral or wild such as Burmese pythons (*Python bivittatus*), originally

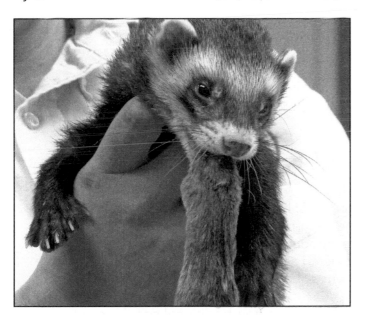

Figure 19-1: The ferret is an example of a domesticated animal. Ferrets are carnivores and while they more commonly eat commercial kibble, the natural diet is whole prey. This practice is adopted by some ferret owners who feed whole animals (such as a mouse here) to their ferrets.

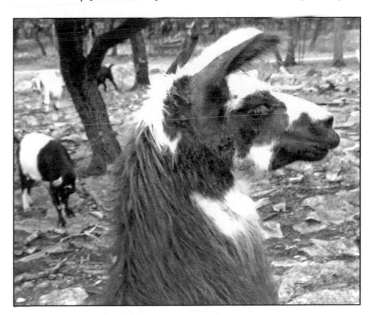

Figure 19-2: A llama is an example of an animal that can exist as domesticated but has escaped and is now free living in the wild (feral).

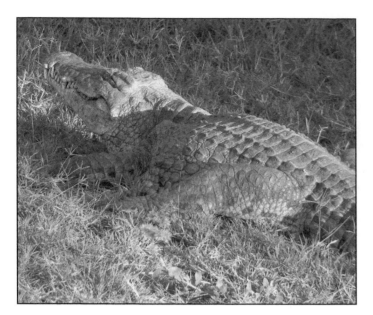

Figure 19-3: Free living non-domesticated animals, such as this crocodile, are truly 'wild'. Wildlife veterinarians and technicians often study these animals in wild habitats (whether that is in a swamp or downtown in a major city).

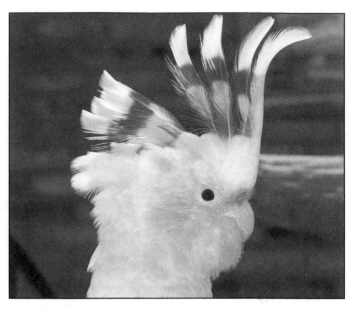

Figure 19-4: While many may consider parrots tame, most are simply captive wild animals. Many parrots, such as this Major Mitchell's cockatoo, are often only a few generations from being wild caught.

from south and southeast Asia, living in Florida **(Figure 19-5)**. A tame animal simply tolerates, accepts or enjoys the presence of humans. Being 'tame' often coincides with domestication. However, many captive wild animals seemingly enjoy human companionship such as green iguanas *(Iguana iguana)*. It should be noted that just because a wild animal, such as a grey squirrel *(Sciurus carolinensis)*, eats out of a person's hand at a park does not equate to being 'tame' **(Figure 19-6)**.

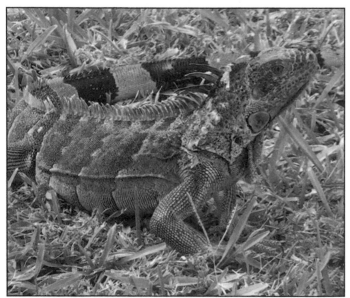

Figure 19-5: Invasive animals are those that live freely in their non-native habitat. For example, green iguanas were introduced to Grand Cayman Island and are now considered a highly invasive species and threaten the existence of other native animals.

It is important to understand these basic definitions because some non-traditional species can turn from seemingly 'tame' to 'wild' inflicting damage upon people, invasive which can affect entire ecosystems or simply be inappropriate for owners who expect the animal to thrive in an unsuitable environment. As the experts in animal care, it is our job to provide accurate information about non-traditional species to protect ourselves, the owners or caretakers, the environment and especially the animal.

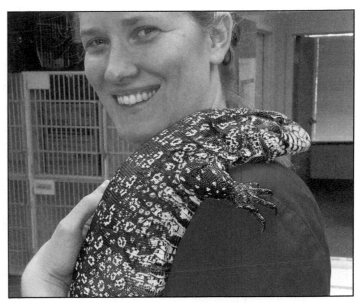

Figure 19-6: Tame animals tolerate, accept or may even enjoy human company. While the term 'tame' often coincides with domestication it is not always the case. This Argentine black and white tegu may seem tame but is far from a domesticated species. Care must be taken when handling all animals, especially non-domestics. It is easy to forget that many non-domestic species are captive wild animals that may unpredictably display wild behaviors.

## Discussion

Caring for non-traditional species can be challenging, exciting and most of all rewarding. There is no adequate means to cover all of the roles of the veterinary technician pertinent to non-traditional species in one chapter. In fact, entire books, seminars, websites and on-line courses are dedicated to very specific aspects of veterinary care for exotic animals.

However, the veterinary technician should understand that exotic animal species deserve a complete history, to be handled with respect and receive complete diagnostic and treatment options like any other domestic animal. Just as blood work, radiographs and exploratory surgery can be performed on a dog, the same is generally true of a rat, goldfish, rattlesnake or just about any other animal given the right tools and expertise.

All animals carry infectious diseases, some of which can affect humans (i.e. zoonotic disease) and other animals of the same or different species. Non-traditional species are no different. However, their infectious diseases may be less commonly known to the general public and to veterinary staff unfamiliar with the animal. Prior to handling exotic animal species, the veterinary technician and team should familiarize themselves with common infectious diseases of that species. Knowledge of these diseases helps the veterinary team determine how best to handle the animal, protect themselves and caretakers and prevent spread to other animals including those in the local environment.

Several references pertaining to non-traditional species are listed at the end of this laboratory assignment. This list is in no way comprehensive and only serves to make you aware that such references are available. However, one reference dedicated to the care of numerous exotic animal species deserves special mention. LafeberVet.com is freely available to veterinary professionals and is a great resource for complete and concise information. Veterinary technicians are encouraged to explore and use the website.

## Handling (Restraint)

Possibly the most important step to physically assessing an animal begins with proper physical restraint **(Figure 19-7)**. This is especially true with exotic animals for numerous reasons:

1. How you handle an animal makes a big impression on the owner or caretaker. Rough or inappropriate handling is a common reason animal caretakers seek advice elsewhere.

2. Poor handling techniques can result in patient stress, altered lab values and injury including adverse behavioral affects that can worsen with each visit. This is commonly seen in pet birds that develop escalating fear responses upon repeat visits.

3. Properly handled animals allow for more complete physical examination and collection of diagnostic samples. This is often essential to establish the health status of the animal.

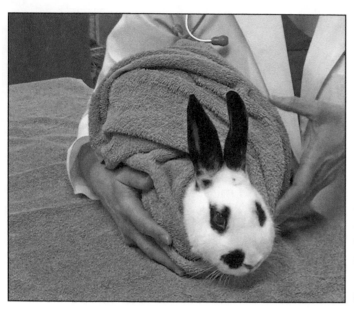

Figure 19-7: Proper handling technique is essential to good veterinary care. Rough or inappropriate handling can result in both physical and behavioral injury to the animal, stress to the owner and damage to the handler(s). This rabbit is safely secured in a towel to prevent the rabbit from suddenly jumping forward which sometimes results in back fractures.

## Proper handling techniques should result in the following:

1. Minimal patient stress considering the situation (Figure 19-8).

2. No injuries to humans or the animal. This includes the spread of disease between animals and people resulting from mechanical transmission associated with handling.

3. A comprehensive physical examination and diagnostic sample collection in a timely fashion.

4. Return to the caretaker, transport device, hospitalization cage, tank or pen, or back into the wild with minimal alteration in behavior, physical attributes or other danger to the animal.

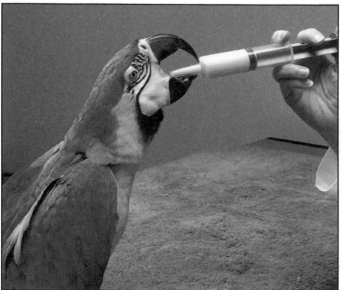

Figure 19-8: Proper handling should allow one to perform a thorough physical examination, collect some non-invasive diagnostic samples, administer medications and return the patient to its owner, traveling cage or natural environment with minimal stress and no injuries to all involved. Proper handling can also foster a good doctor/staff-client-patient relationship. Some animals, such as this blue and gold macaw freely accepting a syringe full of medicated food, may even tolerate some procedures with no or minimal restraint.

Sedation or full anesthesia may be needed to properly restrain exotic animal species (**Figure 19-9**). This is especially true of fractious, nervous, dangerous and highly stressed animals. Special tools may be needed to allow for proper handling and protection. For example, birds of prey (owls, hawks, etc.) are often handled with leather gauntlets (gloves) to prevent talon injuries to the handler. Protective gear may also be used to prevent transmission of disease to or from the animals. For example, some primates should only be handled by staff wearing a surgical gown, mask and gloves and not showing any symptoms of the flu or other common infectious human diseases. The environmental temperature, lighting or even your gloved hands may need to be adjusted prior to holding some species. Wetted surgical gloves washed free of any talc are worn when handling aquatic amphibians (frogs, salamanders, etc.) (**Figure 19-10**).

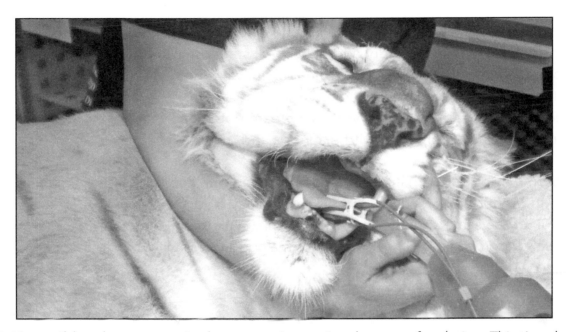

Figure 19-9: Many wild or dangerous animals may require varying degrees of sedation. This tiger had to be fully anesthetized to perform a physical examination, diagnostic sample collection and ultimately a dental cleaning.

Figure 19-10: Some animals, like most aquatic species, require talc free and wetted surgical gloves to prevent damage and microorganism transfer to their delicate skin. As shown with this koi, aquatic animals may need to be examined either in their own environment or in a bucket filled with their tank's water. A supplemental pump, tubing and air stone are often brought along to ensure proper aeration of the traveling fish bucket.

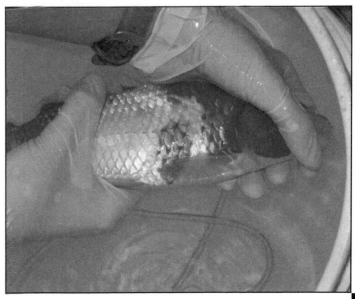

# Husbandry and Behavior

While handling is most important when physically examining animals and collecting samples, understanding husbandry and behavior is equally important to assessing health. Each non-traditional animal species relies on a proper diet, environment and behaviors for normal health. Deviation from normal in any of these parameters commonly results in disease.

By understanding what is normal for the species, the veterinary care team can better determine when something in the animal's care is incorrect and how it may relate to a specific problem. For example, a Syrian hamster (*Mesocricetus auratus*) with infectious diarrhea may need to be treated for the infection but also have a poor diet and dirty, crowded cage corrected. Without addressing the underlying behavioral, dietary or environmental deficits and only treating the obvious problem, the veterinary care team can miss the underlying issue and be faced with a recurring health issue.

The veterinary technician serves a vital role in collecting information about the presenting complaint and the animal's husbandry and behavioral status. It is important to know which questions to ask, so veterinary technicians should familiarize themselves with the presenting animal and the normal husbandry and behavior for that species. This basic information collected on the exotic animal patient helps the veterinary team determine the root cause of the presenting complaint and how best to proceed with diagnosis and treatment.

This information may also determine how best to proceed with handling. For example, a poorly socialized hooded rat (*Rattus norvegicus*) from a lab setting may be difficult to handle or may even bite. The pet version of the same species often requires minimal restraint and rarely bites **(Figure 19-11)**. In either case, without proper handling, no samples may be successfully collected, or data gathered.

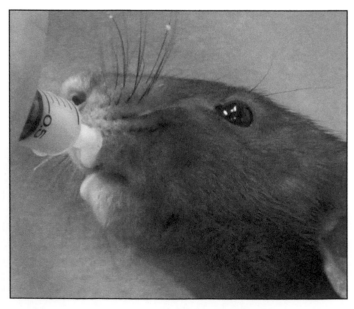

Figure 19-11: Socialized pets may react very differently from their un-socialized counterparts. For example, pet rats are very gentle and can easily be handled and treated as shown here. Laboratory rats are often not accustomed to handling, are more difficult to restrain and may even bite.

# Obtaining Objective Data

With the expertise and correct tools just about any diagnostic test can be completed on non-traditional species. Prior to handling the animal, the veterinary technician should observe the animal and record any data possible. This may include weighing the animal in a carrier, bag, tank, box or other transport device (weigh the device without the animal to obtain patient weight), observing for gait, behavior and topical abnormalities (hair loss, open wounds, etc.) and collecting any other data non-invasively (respiration rate, basic mentation, etc.).

Depending on the patient and the veterinary technician's experience, some exotic animals may be safely handled and allow basic hands-on data collection. This may include recording weight, heart rate, body temperature, collecting stool samples (often from within the carrier) and more. Some animals may also tolerate basic sample collection with minimal restraint such as collecting lice off chickens *(Gallus gallus domesticus)* or ear mites via ear swab from ferrets *(Mustela putorius furo)*. Understanding the basic medical care of exotic species is important. For example, rectal temperatures are not typically taken on reptile, fish, amphibian, and bird species!

Fractious, dangerous and frightened animals often require at least proper restraint if not sedation or anesthesia to collect objective data. The same is often true when collecting invasive diagnostics such as blood, urine, skin scrapings and more.

Of course, sample collection sites and techniques are highly variable between species. For example, blood may be collected easily from the right jugular vein of an umbrella cockatoo *(Cacatua alba)* while cardiocentesis (heart sample collection) would be more appropriate with a corn snake *(Pantherophis guttatus)* and the caudal tail vein could be used with a nurse shark *(Ginglymostoma cirratum)*.

## Administering Medications

In most exotic animal species, the options for delivering medications are the same or similar as with domestic animals. Potential administration routes include oral, transdermal, topical, subcutaneous, intramuscular, intravenous, ophthalmic, aural and more **(Figure 19-12)**.

Species anatomic and physiologic differences help determine how medications are best given. Instead of pilling a Siberian tiger *(Panthera tigris altaica)* with an oral antibiotic, it is often safer (for all involved) to simply hide it in the food. A North African hedgehog *(Atelerix algirus)* with a skin disease will not readily tolerate bathing or application of topical medications and a systemic oral

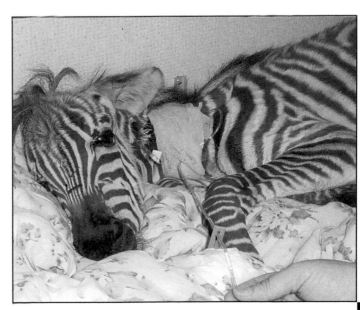

Figure 19-12: Exotic animal species deserve the same level of care as domestics. However, adjustments may need to be made depending on the animal's anatomy, physiology and behavior. Some exotics, like this young zebra receiving intravenous fluids, may be treated just like their domestic counterparts.

drug may be needed. Because of blood flow relating to the renal portal system in reptiles and birds, injectable drugs given in the caudal half of the body of a leopard tortoise *(Stigmochelys pardalis)* may concentrate in the kidneys and contribute to or cause renal disease. For this reason, injectable drugs are given in the front half of the body of most reptiles and birds.

Another consideration is the experience of the person (including the veterinary technician team and the animal caretaker) giving the medication. Risk to the animal and handler should be minimized by proper restraint when giving medications. Recommended treatment protocols that are not safe should be revised. In part it is the veterinary technician's job to ensure that he or she and/or the caretaker are comfortable and competent to safely administer recommended treatments. If not, the prescribing veterinarian should be notified so that an acceptable alternative can be considered.

## Fluid Therapy

Fluid therapy is commonly used in avian and exotic animal medicine. In fact, non-traditional species are often presented in various stages of dehydration.

The route of fluid therapy administration is best determined by the anatomy and physiologic needs of the species in question. However, some generalizations can be made.

Oral fluids are generally used for mild dehydration in patients that are not regurgitating, fully conscious, have control of their swallow reflex and have minimal or no gastrointestinal disease. For example, a friendly guinea pig *(Cavia porcellus)* may readily take syringe fed water but refuse to drink from a bowl.

Subcutaneous fluids can be used in animals that have mild to moderate dehydration. Absorption of subcutaneous fluids is partly dependent upon normal circulatory function and having adequate blood proteins. Subcutaneous fluids are commonly administered to many exotic species especially birds **(Figure 19-13)**.

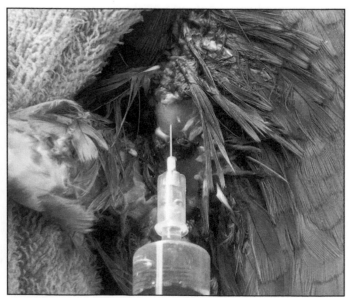

Figure 19-13: As many exotic species successfully hide symptoms of illness, they often present with more advanced diseases than seen on average with domestics. As a result, dehydration is common with sick exotics. Fluid therapy may include intravenous, intraosseous, subcutaneous, oral, intra-abdominal, topical and intraceolomic routes. Inguinal subcutaneous fluids are being administered to an Amazon parrot here.

Intravenous and intraossesous (in the bone) fluids are reserved for more advanced stages of dehydration. These fluid routes may also be used during routine surgeries. Intravenous catheters can be placed anywhere a superficial vein is present and large enough to take the catheter. Intraossesous catheters are commonly placed in small exotic species that have small peripheral veins.

Intracoelomic and Intra-abdominal fluids may also be used with more advanced dehydration or when intravenous, intraossesous and subcutaneous fluids cannot be easily given. Animals without a diaphragm (birds, fish, amphibians, reptiles) have a coelom instead of a thorax and abdomen (mammals). Intraceolomic and intra-abdominal fluids may be administered directly through the skin or during surgery when the belly has been surgically exposed. It should be noted that intracoelomic fluids given to some species, such as birds, may result in dangerous flooding of the respiratory system and should be carefully administered.

Topical fluids should also be mentioned as this route is important for amphibians and fish. Topical fluids include the animal's environment as well as any additional fluids dripped directly on the animal. Water quality is extremely important for aquatic species. The same is true for any fluids dripped on an aquatic animal. Topical fluids should be balanced for pH, osmolality and free of potential toxins prior to application. For example, some salt water fish are temporarily placed in a fresh water solution for a short period of time to treat topical parasites. However, long term exposure can result in death to the fish.

# Performing Diagnostic Tests

Just about any diagnostic test performed on domestic animals can be applied, sometimes with modification, to exotic species.

Blood and fluid based, diagnostics (complete blood counts, serum chemistries, joint tap analysis, cytology, etc.) are commonly performed on exotic species. Because some of our exotic patients are small, reduced sample size can be a limiting factor. Always consult your reference or in-house lab to determine the minimum sample size needed to complete a test. Newer diagnostic machines often run off minute quantities of blood and other samples.

Imaging studies including radiographs, ultrasound, computed tomography, magnetic resonance imaging and more are also commonly used **(Figure 19-14)**. The same limitations that affect domestic animals are also found with exotics. For example, ultrasound does not penetrate air filled cavities (lungs, air sacs, gas-filled intestines). Because birds normally have a well-developed air sac system, ultrasound may have limited use in a healthy mallard (*Anas platyrhynchos*).

Microbiologic assays are performed using aseptic techniques as described for domestic animals. Care should be taken when collecting microbiologic samples from sources that are contaminated from the surrounding environment. For example, cultures of gill specimens from a koi (*Cyprinus carpio*) may reflect the water quality more than organisms affecting the fish **(Figure 19-15)**.

Just about any diagnostic test performed on domestic species can be completed on non-domestics. The main limitations often are animal anatomy and physiology, expertise of the person/people collecting the sample and sometimes requirements of the diagnostic test.

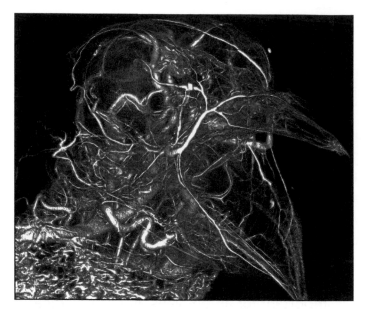

**Figure 19-14:** Advanced imaging such as high detailed radiographs, computed tomography (AKA CT) and magnetic resonance imaging (AKA MRI) can often be performed on exotic animal species. This is a detailed contrast arteriovenogram CT image of a pigeon head. Picture courtesy of Scarlet Imaging, LLC, www.scarletimaging.com.

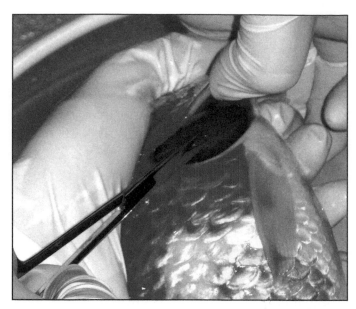

**Figure 19-15:** Diagnostic samples from exotics can also give us information about the animal's environment and living conditions. Gill biopsies in fish may reveal infectious agents and some disease states but also tell attending veterinarians a lot about the water quality in the animal's environment.

# Anesthesia and Analgesia

Anesthetics are commonly used in non-traditional species. Some animals must be anesthetized just to complete an exam and collect diagnostic samples. Anesthetics may be topical, injectable or inhaled and may be used for local, regional or systemic anesthesia. Because the nervous system of non-mammalian animals is often quite unlike that of mammalian species, entirely different classes of drugs may be used as anesthetics. For example, Tricaine methanesulfonate (more commonly known as MS-222) is commonly used to anesthetize frogs and fish placed in a medicated water bath.

Animals undergoing anesthetic procedures deserve careful monitoring. In fact, monitoring vitals and adjusting anesthetic depth is often more intensive with avian and exotic species compared to that which is done with most domestics. Common equipment such as electrocardiogram (ECG), pulse oximetry, capnography and more can also be used in exotic species. Also, physical changes associated with depth of anesthesia (respiratory rate, eye position, heart rate, mucus membrane color, etc.) can also be monitored in anesthetized exotic patients.

Avian and exotic species clearly experience pain and often need analgesics. However, because of the basic nature of many non-traditional species to hide signs of illness, we may not as readily recognize pain or distress in these animals. It is important that animals undergoing painful procedures or sustaining significant injuries, should receive appropriate analgesics **(Figure 19-16)**. Understanding the behavior of these animals can help to determine if stress or pain is present.

Because we don't have as many studies involving the use of anesthetics and analgesics in exotic species as we do in domestic animals, these drugs should be used carefully in non-traditional species. While safe in some domestic animals, some drugs are extremely toxic to exotic species.

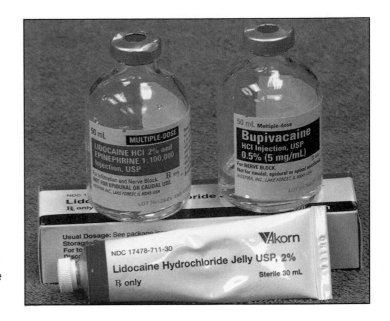

Figure 19-16: Local, regional and systemic analgesics should be used as needed for any animal in pain. The same is true with exotic animals.

For example, the common non-steroidal anti-inflammatory drug diclofenac used in cattle is extremely toxic to *Gyps* genus vultures rapidly resulting in kidney failure and death. Drug types and doses should be carefully checked with current and reputable resources that focus on avian and exotic species.

## Risks of Keeping Non-Traditional Species as Pets

Keeping non-traditional species is not without risks. Not only may keeping some of these animals be dangerous to the owner, but the animals may also pose a danger to the environment (invasive species) and other animals (trauma, infectious diseases and more). Additionally, some animals (including most native species) are illegal to own without proper permits.

Because we are often presented with sick exotic species, we should consider that these non-traditional animals may carry atypical diseases that can affect more than just the patient. For example, Gambian pouched rats (*Cricetomys gambianus*) and prairie dogs (genus *Cynomys*) have been listed on the Centers for Disease Control (CDC) website because they can carry monkey pox that has affected numerous people in several states. It is important to use basic sanitation when handling all animals. Some species such as primates often require more precautions (gowns, gloves, masks) because of real risks of disease transmission to and from these animals. Herpes B virus found in some primates is often fatal to humans. This is an obvious serious concern encountered when handling macaques (genus *Macaca*) of which 80 to 90% may be infected. Those involved with the care of exotic species should be familiar with common risks associated with handling the animal and its tissues and take appropriate precautions.

Some exotics are extremely dangerous to handle because they can inflict serious injury to humans **(Figure 19-17)**. Obviously venomous animals and exotic carnivores (such as lions) are dangerous. Even the common iguana (*Iguana iguana*) can inflict nasty bites when provoked. Large animals (camels, deer and other hoof stock) may be difficult to handle and cause serious injury without appropriate restraint, sedation, equipment and experience. In general, it is best to understand the animal's basic features (teeth, claws, etc.) and behavior and your own limitations before handling exotic species.

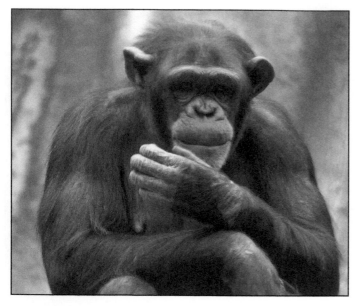

**Figure 19-17:** Some exotic species can be extremely dangerous by inflicting life-threatening injuries or carrying highly infectious diseases that are deadly to humans and other animals. Chimpanzees are highly intelligent and incredibly strong. They also carry diseases that can be shared with humans putting both species at risk.

Many non-traditional species are illegal to own. Ownership of some exotic species is restricted by state, federal and even international laws to help prevent illegal trade, establishing invasive feral colonies, danger to the public and other reasons. For example, ownership of Quaker parakeets (*Myiopsitta monachus*) is restricted or illegal in many US states because of their ability to establish feral colonies. It is important to understand local, state and federal laws pertaining to exotic animal ownership to help protect the owners and the animals.

# LAB 19: WORKSHEET

Name/Group Name:_____

Date:_____

Using your web based and book resources, answer the following questions:

1. A red eared slider (*Trachemys scripta elegans*) comes into your clinic and has been diagnosed with an aural abscess. What is this and in general terms, what is needed to diagnose and treat the condition?_____

_____

_____

_____

2. A cockatiel (*Nymphicus hollandicus*) comes into the clinic where you are working and is diagnosed with psittacosis. What is this and why is it important that the owners and veterinary staff understand this disease?_____

_____

_____

_____

3. A domestic chicken (*Gallus gallus domesticus*) is necropsied and Marek's disease is suspected. The chicken comes from a backyard flock of birds. Is this disease a concern for the other chickens and people handling the chickens?_____

_____

_____

_____

4. An apparently healthy rabbit (*Oryctolagus cuniculus*) comes in for a routine exam, blood work and urine. Where would you collect blood from a rabbit?_____

_____

_____

_____

5. Parsley is high in oxalic acid. Why would this be a concern with guinea pigs (*Cavia porcellus*)?

_____

_____

_____

_____

6. You are working on a large bearded dragon (*Pogona vitticeps*) that is anorexic, depressed and dehydrated. Where can you collect blood from this lizard? What tests do you anticipate the veterinarian will order and therefore what collection devices do you need?_____

_____

_____

_____

7. A Pekin duck (*Anas platyrhynchos*) presents to your hospital with a fractured wing. What analgesics can be used safely and effectively with this duck? Will the fracture and/or analgesics influence a CBC (if ordered)?_____

_____

_____

_____

8. A client calls about a raccoon (*Procyon lotor*) that is showing neurological signs (wobbly gait and erratic behavior). You immediately tell the owner to contact animal control and to stay away from the raccoon because of concern about what major disease?_____

_____

9. A ferret (*Mustela putorius furo*) presents for a routine exam and vaccinations. What is the most common concern with vaccines and ferrets that owners should understand prior to vaccination?

_____

10. A client finds and keeps a desert tortoise (*Gopherus agassizii*) while traveling in the southwest United States. Is it legal to keep these? If not, why not?_____

_____

_____

_____

# REFERENCES

There are too many good references on non-traditional species medicine, biology and general care to mention here. The following list is limited and only intended to give students a starting point from which to explore avian and exotic animal care. Many lay and professional journals, organizational and other resources are available for those interested in learning about and working with unique species.

## Websites

1. General pet avian and exotic animal information: www.Lafebervet.com

2. Wildlife, Exotic Pets, and Emerging Zoonoses: http://wwwnc.cdc.gov/eid/article/13/1/06-0480_article

3. General biology information: http://www.wikipedia.org/

## Books

1. Carpenter JW. Exotic Animal Formulary (5th Ed). Elsevier, 2018.

2. Fowler MF. Restraint and Handling of Wild and Domestic Animals (3rd Ed). Wiley-Blackwell, 2008.

3. Fox JG, Anderson LC, Loew FM, Quimby FW. Laboratory Animal Medicine (2nd Ed). Academic Press. 2002.

4. Harrison GJ, Lightfoot TL. Clinical Avian Medicine Volumes I and II. Spix Publishing, 2006.

5. Mader DR. Reptile Medicine and Surgery (2nd Ed). Elsevier, 2005.

6. Mader DR, Diver SJ. Current Therapy in Reptile Medicine and Surgery. Elsevier, 2014.

7. Miller RE, Fowler MF. Fowler's Zoo and Wild Animal Medicine Current Therapy (7th Ed). Elsevier, 2012.

8. Speer BL. Current Therapy in Avian Medicine and Surgery. Elsevier, 2016.

9. Quesenberry KE, Carpenter JW. Ferrets, Rabbits and Rodents (3rd Ed). Elsevier, 2012.

10. Stoskopf M. Fish Medicine Volumes I and II (2nd Ed). ART Sciences LC, 2010.

11. Veterinary Clinics of North America: Exotic Animal Practice. Elsevier.

12. Wright KM, Whitaker BR. Amphibian Medicine and Captive Husbandry. Krieger Publishing Company, 2001.

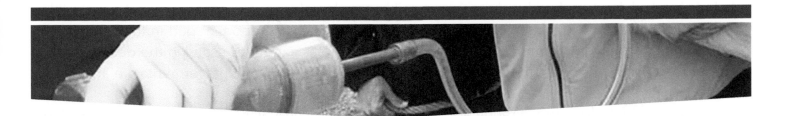

# CHAPTER 20

## RUMEN FLUID COLLECTION AND EVALUATION

# OBJECTIVES

This lab serves to introduce technicians to a technique that is often performed on cattle to assess rumen function and therefore gastrointestinal health. The collection of rumen fluid and subsequent analysis is a task best undertaken by someone with a working knowledge of rumen anatomy and the associated physiological impact. Because the rumen plays such an important part in the overall nutritional status of ruminant animals, the analysis of its contents is extremely useful in the determination of what may or may not be occurring within the organ which is known for its fermentative abilities.

The AVMA-CVTEA does not directly address rumen fluid testing within the Veterinary Technician Student Essential and Recommended Skills List, however there are several areas in which the proficiency gained within this lab will stand the technician in good stead. These areas include the ability to:

√ Properly carry out analysis of laboratory specimens
√ Prepare specimens for diagnostic analysis
√ Perform microbiological procedures and evaluations to include
  • Collection of representative samples

Although the guidelines are not specific in terms of addressing rumen fluid collection, students will be able to appreciate the need to understand and be proficient in the laboratory regardless of the specimen with which they are presented.

# KEY TERMS

| | | |
|---|---|---|
| Anorexia | Fermentation | Phosphate |
| Bicarbonate | Frick's Speculum | Putrefaction |
| Bloat | Lactic Acidosis | Silage |
| Buffers | Ororuminal | Transfaunation |
| Concentrate | pH | Viscosity |

# INTRODUCTION

The rumen is part of a multi-compartmentalized gastrointestinal system found in ruminant animals (cattle, sheep, goat, deer, and giraffe). The ruminant stomach may be divided into two parts; the fore stomach and the true stomach. The fore stomach is made up of three compartments, the rumen, reticulum and omasum. The true stomach is called the abomasum. The fore stomach is responsible for the fermentation of feed for further digestion and contains multiple types of microorganisms. These microorganisms call the rumen fluid "home" and it is this fluid that is collected and examined for evaluation of gastrointestinal health.

## Discussion

Ororuminal collection involves the passage of a tube into the rumen to retrieve the rumen fluid. Although this procedure can be aseptically difficult, care should be taken at all times to avoid salivary contamination due to the use of buffers which enhance saliva. Contamination with these buffers will contribute to erroneous results, especially with regard to bicarbonate or phosphate determination.

There are several testing methods that are important when assessing rumen fluid; some are physical observations while others are more biochemical or microbiological in nature. A good, basic understanding of microbiological handling and testing techniques will be helpful (See Chapters 12 and 13).

## Color, Odor and Consistency – Physical Findings

Physical characteristics such as color, odor and fluid consistency (i.e. viscosity) should be noted immediately upon collection **(Figure 20-1)**. This, entails smelling and visual inspection of the fluid. While these tests are somewhat subjective, they do provide information about dietary habits and gastrointestinal function. **Table 20-1** lists some expected findings and their implications.

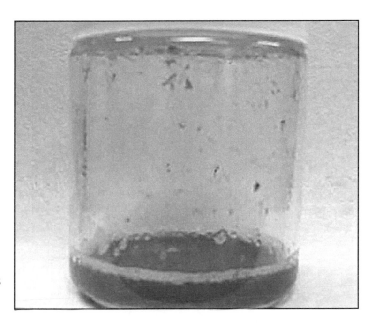

Figure 20-1: As soon as rumen fluid is collected evaluate and record the physical characteristics such as color, odor and fluid consistency (i.e. viscosity).

## pH Determinations

The pH of the rumen contents determines whether or not a fluid is alkaline (basic) or acidic (acid based) and the types of organisms that may be able to survive in that environment **(Figure 20-2)**. This is very important to ruminant physiology because certain microorganisms are needed to break down feed for digestion. If the feed is not broken down appropriately, animals cannot reap the nutritional benefit needed for continued good health.

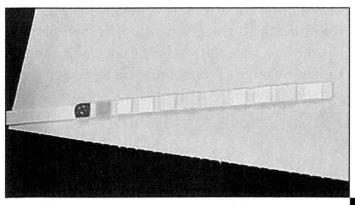

Figure 20-2: A simple pH strip rapidly allows one to determine whether rumen fluid is acidic or basic. This information helps clinicians understand what type of organisms can live in the given environment.

## TABLE 20-1
## Rumen Fluid POC References

| COLOR | REASONING |
|---|---|
| Yellow/brown: | Corn silage/straw diet |
| Brown/olive: | Concentrate diet |
| Green: | Pasture diet |
| Milky gray/brown: | Lactic acidosis |
| | |
| **ODOR** | **REASONING** |
| Aromatic: | Normal |
| Acidic/sour: | Lactic acidosis |
| Rotting: | Rumen putrification/infection |
| | |
| **CONSISTENCY** | **REASONING** |
| Excess viscosity: | High saliva content |
| Watery, few particles: | Anorexic |
| Bubbles: | Bloat |
| | |
| **pH** | **INTERPRETATION** |
| 8 and above: | Saliva contamination, putrification |
| 7 to 8: | Reduced feed intake |
| 6 to 7: | Normal pH of cattle |
| 5 to 5.6 | High grain diet or pasture fed/early lactic acidosis |
| 5.5 | Lactic acidosis |
| | |
| **METHYLENE BLUE REDUCTION TEST TIME** | **INTERPRETATION** |
| 3 to 6 minutes: | Adequate bacteria are present |
| 10+ minutes: | Inadequate bacteria are present |

# Bacterial Assessments

There are a variety of tests for examination and assessment of micro-organisms in rumen fluid **(Figure 20-3)**. The presence of certain organisms confirms that the associated biochemical reactions are occurring. In other cases, the ability of the microbes to break down feed (through biochemical reactions) must be tested to determine if the appropriate biochemical reactions are occurring. With most biochemical tests, careful attention is required during the test procedure to ensure proper results.

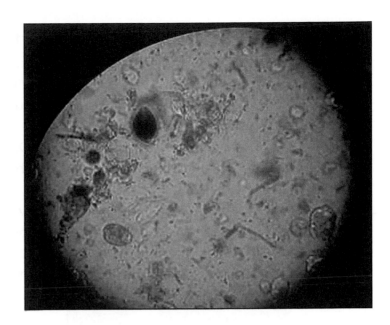

Figure 20-3: Several tests can be used to assess the microorganisms present in rumen fluid. One of the easiest is light microscopy. Microscopy allows one to quickly see numbers, types and motility of rumen organisms.

## CONCLUSION
Veterinary technicians possess the knowledge and organizational skills to render themselves irreplaceable within a large animal clinic/operation. With the tools learned in this lab, technicians add one more weapon to their arsenal that clinicians rely on frequently when considering rumen health.

# LAB 20
# RUMEN FLUID COLLECTION AND EVALUATION

## INTRODUCTION
Rumen fluid collection and testing are often needed when ruminant animals are "off their feed" or otherwise in gastric compromise. Careful, aseptic collection of rumen fluids will aid in a diagnosis so that swift treatment can be initiated. It should be noted that gastric distress can quickly turn deadly and time is of the essence.

## EQUIPMENT LIST
1. Frick's speculum
2. Large animal stomach tube
3. Halter and rope
4. Dosing syringe
5. Sterile plastic container with lid

## LAB ASSIGNMENT
This lab is designed to acquaint students with the correct protocol for collecting rumen fluid and to enhance their ability to perform point-of-care (POC) testing. Laboratory analysis provides results from which a clinician can formulate a successful plan of treatment. Students should work in pairs or larger groups according to how much rumen fluid is collected, so that all tests may be conducted and observed by the entire class. Findings are recorded on the results page and submitted according to the instructor's directions at the completion of lab.

# Collection of Rumen Fluid (cattle)

Cows should be safely restrained within a chute and head gate with a halter and lead rope securely fitted **(Figure 20-4)**. While the head is securely immobilized, a Frick's Speculum should be utilized. The handler who is inserting the speculum should stand close to the cow, wrapping an arm around the top of the neck to reach over in such a way as to hold the head steady and open the mouth while simultaneously inserting the speculum. Once the speculum is inserted into the esophagus, you will hear gurgling noises emanating from the metal tube. Pass the tube through the speculum and down the esophagus. To assist in passage, blow into the tube to aid in dilation of the esophagus. If placed correctly you will see movement of the tube in the esophagus, smell grass or fermented gases emanating from the tube or while blowing air into the tube and listening for gurgling sounds. If the animal begins to cough or wheeze, the tube has been misplaced into the trachea (similar to surgical intubation) and must be withdrawn and reinserted.

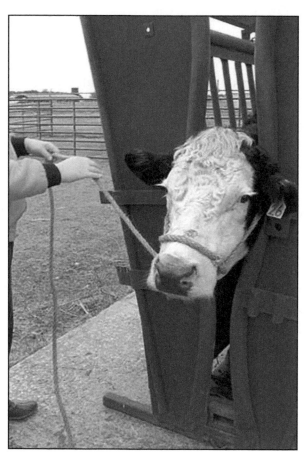

Figure 20-4: In preparation for rumen fluid collection, the cow should be secured in an appropriately sized chute with halter and lead rope securely fitted.

Once the tube has been placed, rumen fluid may be extracted by kinking the tube and simultaneously withdrawing it, therefore trapping a small amount of fluid in the end of the tube. A dosing syringe can also be attached to the tube to collect a larger amount of fluid before withdrawing the tube **(Figure 20-5)**. It is important to discard the first 200 mL of rumen fluid as it is most likely contaminated. An assistant should be standing at the ready with a sterile container to drain fluid into as the tube is withdrawn from the cow **(Figure 20-6)**. The container lid should be firmly closed to avoid further contamination. All POC testing should be carried out immediately. The laboratory testing should be completed as quickly as possible upon returning to the lab. Be advised that the microbes that exist within rumen fluid will die very quickly outside of their natural habitat, this is especially important when attempting to gauge microbial function. Do not expose the sample to extreme temperature changes such as sitting the container on a cool bench or tabletop.

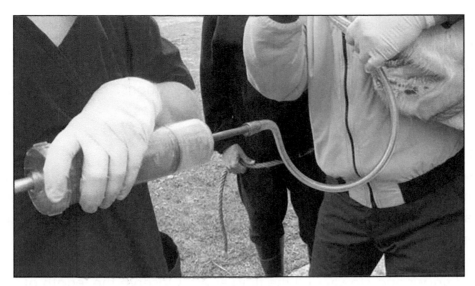

Figure 20-5: Once the Rumen tube has been properly placed, the external end of the tube can be kinked and pulled out. This action will trap the rumen fluid in the internal end of the tube. Alternatively, as shown here, a dosing syringe can be attached to the external end of the tube and a larger sample of rumen fluid can then be collected.

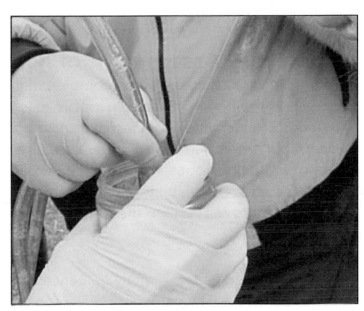

Figure 20-6: Once the rumen fluid has been collected, either in the tube and/or in the dosing syringe, discard the first 200 mls which is commonly contaminated. Use a sterile container to collect the remaining rumen specimen and store securely for further analysis. Perform laboratory diagnostics as quickly as possible.

## Assessment of Physical Characteristics

Physical characteristics including color, odor and consistency should be noted and recorded imme-diately upon collection. This is easily done cow-side through the use of the technician's senses.

## Color:

Through visual inspection, it is possible to ascertain the color of the rumen fluid which in turn aids in evaluation of the animal's diet. To most accurately describe the fluid color, examine it in a strong light within a clear container to avoid variations due to opacity, lack of transparency, etc. **Table 20-1:** Rumen Fluid POC Reference lists the most common colors and the type of diet these are associated with.

## Odor:

The odor of rumen fluid despite its origin should be pleasant and non-offensive. Typically, the odor is described as aromatic, acidic/sour or rotting; each description is indicative of certain physiological and biochemical activities which are taking place in the rumen. In order to "smell" fluids in an aseptic manner (avoiding contamination of fluids as well as yourself) hold the container out from your nose and waft fumes towards you. Record your observations. **Table 20-1:** Rumen Fluid POC Reference lists the odors along with their most probable causes.

## Consistency:

Consistency is also known as viscosity which is a physical quality of a liquid describing the degree of thickness or smoothness observed. The consistency of rumen fluid while somewhat subjective, is indicative of dietary habits, saliva production and some conditions of distress in ruminants such as "Bloat". Consistency is easily measured by performing the 'pull test'. This is done (wearing gloves) by pipetting a small amount of rumen fluid onto your second finger, then place your thumb on top of your second finger and slowly pull the fluid apart. Observe the length of the string, if there is little to no stringing between the fingers before breakage, it is recorded as "low viscosity", if there is stringing, the sample is regarded as "highly" or "excessively viscous". **Table 20-1:** Rumen Fluid POC Reference lists the most common causes of differences which may be observed in the viscosity of rumen fluid.

# Laboratory Assessment of Rumen Fluid and Microbial Populations

Laboratory assessments may be completed on the rumen fluid to assess the environment of the fluid within the rumen. It is also possible to examine the actual microbial life in the fluid if it is done quickly. It should be noted that the microbes which reside within the rumen are extremely susceptible to temperature change, excessive light and time spent outside of the rumen. Assessment of rumen microbes and the rumen environment is important for diagnostic purposes and to determine microbial viability when considering the transfer of rumen fluid from one cow to another in an attempt to repopulate the rumen with healthy microbial life (transfaunation).

## pH:

The pH of rumen fluid is directly influenced by the animal's diet; grain-fed cattle generally exhibit a pH of 5.5 to 6.5 while animals on a green fodder diet will have a pH range of 6 to7. The pH of rumen fluid also influences the ability of microbes to digest and therefore must be maintained in a consistent manner. Changes in pH can effect the ability to digest certain substances, particularly fiber by fibrolytic bacteria which are extremely sensitive to changes in pH levels.

The pH is easily checked with the use of litmus paper or even the pH strip portion of a urinalysis strip by placing a drop of fluid on the paper and reading the color change according to the color chart. **Table 20-1:** Rumen Fluid POC Reference lists the interpretations which may be drawn from a variety of pH readings as to the state of the rumen and its contents.

## Methylene Blue Reduction Test:

This test is performed to gauge the effectiveness of microbial activity in the rumen. Although the test is routinely completed in the laboratory, it may be done as a POC activity as it only requires Methylene Blue stain, rumen fluid and a timer. The test requires preparation of a test tube by adding .5 mL of a .03% solution (.03 mL Methylene Blue stain dissolved in 99.97 mL of water), then add 10 mL of fresh rumen fluid and set the timer (add the rumen fluid to the stain). If the stain is added to the rumen fluid the test may not be successful. Note the amount of time that it takes for the rumen microbes to decolorize the solution. The normal time is roughly 3 to 6 minutes. **Table 20-1:** Rumen Fluid POC Reference lists the interpretation of the time that it takes for the fluid to be cleared of the methyl blue stain.

## Protozoal Motility Assessment:

In addition to the presence of microbes in the rumen fluid, it is important to assess the motility of any protozoan inhabitants (i.e. energy levels) in the fluid. Inactive protozoa are not normally functional. Although this is a somewhat subjective, yes or no answer (Are the protozoa moving?); it is important information for the assessment of rumen health. The assessment is completed by placing a drop of fresh rumen fluid on a slide and adding a drop of Lugol's Iodine. Those protozoans which are uniformly stained have healthy energy levels, while those with decreased energy output are not stained as readily. A notation in the medical record should be made regarding the motility (energy level) of protozoans in the rumen.

## Bacteria Identification:

Bacteria may be identified as cocci or bacilli by performing a Gram Stain of the rumen fluid. If the animal is healthy, the fluid will be predominantly populated with Gram negative bacteria of a heterogeneous nature. If, however, there is a case of lactic acidosis there will be a larger, more uniform population of gram positive bacteria. A note regarding the population of microbes as observed when the fluid is subjected to Gram staining should be made in the medical record. The type of microbe (Gram negative or positive) present will be indicative of the health status of the rumen.

HINTS: Rumen fluid must be handled carefully to preserve the integrity of the microbes.
√ Do not expose the container to drastic temperature changes.
√ Always sit the container on a pad or towel, never directly on a cool counter, this will induce cold shock and kill the microbes before you get started.
√ Shield the rumen fluid from direct sunlight.
√ Run tests immediately, no waiting because the microbes begin to die once out of the anaerobic environment of the rumen.

# LAB RESULTS

Name/Group: _____

Date/Time: _____

Animal ID: _____

Species: _____

Total Amount of Fluid Collected: _____

Color: _____

Odor: _____

Consistency/Viscosity: _____

pH: _____

Methylene Blue Reduction Test: _____

Lugol's Iodine Protozoa Assessment: _____

Gram Stain: _____

Discussion Questions:

1. What is the implication of a lack of uptake of Lugol's Iodine by protozoans, what are some health conditions that may be indicated?

2. Which types of bacteria are normally seen with Gram staining, what are the implications of high Gram negative populations? Gram positive populations? Cocci?

3. Why is Point-of-Care testing important when dealing with rumen fluid. What are some precautions that may be taken to preserve rumen inhabitants until they are transferred back to the laboratory environment?

# REFERENCES

1. Reece, W.O. (2000). Functional Anatomy and Physiology of Domestic Animals, 3rd Ed. Philadelphia, PA: Lippincott, Williams & Wilkins.

2. Anderson, D. E. & Rings, D. M. (2009). Current Veterinary Therapy: Food Animal Practice, 5th Ed. St. Louis, MO: Saunders-Elsevier.

3. Bowen, R. (2009). Rumen Physiology and Rumination. Retrieved from: http://www.vivo.colostate.edu/hbooks/pathphys/digestion/herbivores/rumination.html

4. Bassert, J. M. & McCurnin, D. M. (2010). McCurnin's Clinical Textbook for Veterinary Technicians, 7th Ed. St. Louis, MO: Saunders-Elsevier.

5. Rockett, J. & Bosted, S. (2007). Veterinary Clinical Procedures in Large Animal Practice. Clifton Park, NY: Delmar-Cengage.

# APPENDICES

# APPENDIX A
# PROFICIENCY CHECK-OFF SHEET
# ESSENTIAL AND RECOMMENDED SKILLS
# LABORATORY PROCEDURES

Essential & Recommended Skills                                            Date

1. Proper package, handling & storage of specimens for laboratory analysis  _____

2. Prepare specimens for diagnostic analysis                             _____

3. Select/maintain laboratory equipment                                  _____

4. Implement quality control (GROUP)                                     _____

5. Urinalysis:
   Physical properties (color, clarity, specific gravity, odor)          _____
   Chemical properties testing                                           _____
   Examine and identify sediment                                         _____

6. Complete Blood Count
   Hemoglobin                                                            _____
   Packed Cell Volume (PCV)                                              _____
   Total Protein (TP)                                                    _____
   White Cell Count (WBC)                                                _____
   Red Cell Count (RBC)                                                  _____

7. Examination of blood film
   Prepare blood film and stain                                         _____
   Leukocyte differential                                               _____
   Evaluate erythrocyte morphology                                      _____
   Estimate platelet numbers                                            _____
   Calculate absolute values                                            _____
   Correct white blood cell counts for nucleated cells                  _____

8. Calculate hematological indices                                       _____

9. Coagulation Testing (GROUP) Perform one of the following:
   Buccal mucosal bleeding time                                    _____
   Activated Clotting Time (ACT)                                   _____
   Prothrombin Time (PT)                                           _____
   Partial Thromboplastin Time (PTT)                              _____
   Fibrinogen Assay                                               _____

10. Blood Chemistry Testing (mechanical) Glucose, BUN, Common Enzymes    _____

11. Serologial Testing (ELISA, Slide card agglutination)            _____

12. Microbiological Procedures/Evaluations
    Collect representative sample                                  _____
    Culture bacteria and perform sensitivity testing              _____
    Identify common animal pathogens using commercially available
    media/reagents (GROUP)                                        _____
    Collect milk samples and conduct mastitis testing (GROUP)     _____
    Biochemical testing (GROUP)                                   _____
    Staining procedures commonly seen in microbiology             _____
    Culture and identify common dermatophytes                     _____

13. Cytological Evaluation
    Collect, prepare and evaluate transudate, exudate and cytological specimen    _____
    Perform fine needle aspirates and impression smear preparation    _____
    Prepare and stain bone marrow specimens                       _____
    Collect, prepare and examine ear cytology                     _____
    Collect, prepare and evaluate canine vaginal smears (GROUP)   _____
    Evaluate semen                                                _____
    Understand timing and types of pregnancy testing             _____
    Assist with artificial insemination                           _____

14. Necropsy
    Perform postmortem examination or dissection of non-preserved
    animal (GROUP)                                                _____
    Collect samples, store and ship according to lab protocol (GROUP)    _____
    Explain handling of rabies suspect and sample safety          _____
    Handle disposal of dead animals                               _____
    Perform humane euthanasia procedures                          _____

# APPENDIX B
# NAHRS REPORTABLE DISEASE LIST

| SPECIES | DISEASE | NICKNAME | CAUSATIVE AGENT |
|---|---|---|---|
| Bovine | | | |
| | Foot and Mouth Disease | FMD | Aphthovirus Genus |
| | Vesicular Stomatitis | VS | Visiculovirus Genus |
| | Rinderpest | RP | Morbillivirus Genus |
| | Contagious Bovine Pleuropneumonia | CBP | M. mycoides |
| | Lumpy Skin Disease | LSD | A. bovis |
| | | | A. gerencseriae |
| | Rift Valley Fever | RVF | Phlebovirus Genus |
| | Crimean Congo Hemorrhagic Fever | CCHF | Nairovirus Genus |
| | Bluetongue | The Dancing Disease | Odocoileus virginianus, Antilocapra americana |
| | | | Ovis canadensis |
| | Anthrax | Wool Sorters Disease | B. anthracis |
| | Aujesky's Disease | Pseudorabies, Mad Itch | Varicellovirus Genus |
| | Echinococcus | Hydatidosis | E. granulosus |
| | Cowdriosis | Heartwater | C. ruminantium |
| | Leptospirosis | Weil's Disease | L. interrogans |
| | Q-Fever | Q-Fever | C. burnetii |
| | Rabies | Mad Dog Disease | Lyssaviruses Genus |
| | Paratuberculosis | Johne's Disease | M. avian paratuberculosis |
| | New World Screwworm | NWS | C. hominivorax |
| | Old World Screwworm | OWS | C. bezziana |
| | Anaplasmosis | Gallsickness | A. marginale, A. centrale |
| | Babesiosis | Nantucket Fever | B. bovis, B. bigmina |
| | Bovine Brucellosis | Bang's Disease | B. abortus |
| | Brucellosis | Undulent's Fever | B. melitensis |
| | Swine Brucellosis | Undulent's Fever | B. suis |
| | Bovine Genital Campylobacteriosis | Vibriosis | C. fetus venerealis |
| | Bovine Tuberculosis | Bovine TB | M. bovis |
| | Bovine Viral Disease | BVD | Pestivirus Genus |
| | Enzootic Bovine Leukosis | BLV | T-lymphotropic virus |
| | Hemorrhagic Septicemia | HS | P. multicida |
| | Infectious Bovine Rhinotracheitis | Bovine Herpes | Bovine herpesvirus 1 |
| | Theileriasis | East Coast Fever | T. annulata, T. parva |
| | Trichomoniasis | Trich | T. foetus |
| | Trypanosomiasis | Tsetse Transmitted - TTT | T. congolense, T. vivax, T. brucei, T. evansi |
| | Malignant Catarrhal Fever | MCF | Rhadinovirus Genus |
| | Bovine Spongiform Encephalopathy | Mad Cow Disease (BSE) | Prion |
| | Epizootic Hemorrhagic Disease | EHD | Epizootic Hemorrhagic Disease Virus (EHD) |
| | Bluetongue Virus (BT) | BTV | Bluetongue virus (Orbivirus) |
| Capine/Ovine | | | |
| | Foot and Mouth Disease | FMD | Orbivirus (22 species) |

| | | |
|---|---|---|
| Vesicular Stomatitis | VS | Visiculovirus Genus |
| Rinderpest | Cattle Plague | Morbillivirus Genus |
| Peste des petits ruminants | PPRV | Morbillivirus Genus |
| Rift Valley Fever | Infectious Hepatitis | Phlebovirus genus |
| | | Odocoileus virginianus, |
| | | Antilocapra americana |
| | | Ovis canadensis |
| Bluetongue Virus (BT) | BTV | Bluetongue virus (Orbivirus) |
| Crimean Congo Hemorrhagic Fever | CCHF | Nairovirus genus |
| Sheep pox and goat pox | SPV/GPV | Myxoma viruses |
| Anthrax | Wool Sorters Disease | B. anthracis |
| Aujesky's Disease | Pseudorabies | Varicellovirus Genus |
| Echinococcus | Hydatidosis | E. granulosus |
| Cowdriosis | Heartwater | C. ruminantium |
| Leptospirosis | Weil's Disease | L. interrogans |
| Q-Fever | Q-Fever | C. burnetii |
| Paratuberculosis | Johne's Disease | M. avium paratuberculosis |
| New World Screwworm | Screw-worm | C. hominivorax |
| Old World Screwworm | Screw-worm | C. bezziana |
| Brucellosis | Undulent Fever | B. melitensis |
| Ovine Epididymitis | OE | B. ovis |
| Caprine arthritis/Encephalitis | CAE | Lentivirus Genus |
| Contagious agalactia | CA | M. agalactiae, |
| | | M. putrefaciens, |
| | | M. mycoides |
| | | M. capricolum |
| Contagious Caprine Pleuropneumonia | CCP | M. capricolum |
| | | capripneumoniae |
| Rabies | Mad Dog Disease | Lyssaviruses Genus |
| Bovine Tuberculosis | Bovine TB | M. bovis |
| Enzootic Abortion of Ewe | Chlymidial abortion | O. psittacosis, |
| | | C. Psittaci |
| Nairobi Sheep Disease | NSD | Bunyaviridae |
| Salmonella S. | | S abortusovis |
| Scrapie | TSE | Prion |
| Maedi-visni | Ovine Progressive Pneumonia | Lentiviruses Genus |
| Theilesiasis | Theilesiasis | T. annulata, T. parvis |
| Tularemia | Rabbit Fever | F. tularensis |
| West Nile Fever | WNF/WNV | Flavivirus Genus |

Equine

| | | |
|---|---|---|
| Vesicular Stomatitis | VS | Visiculovirus Genus |
| African Horse Fever | AHF | Orbivirus (9 serotypes) |
| Anthrax | Wool Sorters Disease | B. anthracis |
| Leptospirosis | Weil's Disease | L. interrogans |
| Rabies | Mad Dog Disease | Lyssaviruses Genus |
| New World Screwworm | Screw-worm | C. hominivorax |
| Old World Screwworm | Screw-worm | C. bezziani |
| Trichinella | Trichinosis | T. spiralis |
| Contagious equine metritis | Equine VD | T. equigenitalis |
| Echinococcus | Hydatidosis | E. granulosus |
| Dourine Equine | VD | T. equiperadum |

| | | |
|---|---|---|
| Equine Encephalomyelitis | (Eastern) EEE | EEE Virus |
| Equine Encephalomyelitis | (Western) WEE | WEE Virus |
| Equine Infectious Anemia | EIA | Lentivirus Genus |
| Equine Influenza Type A | Horse Flu | Orthomyxovirus (New Zealand) |
| Equine Piroplasmosis | Babesiosis | B. equi, B. caballi |
| Equine Rhinopneumonitis | Equine Herpesvirus | Influenza Virus A |
| Equine Herpesvirus myeloencephalopathy | EHV-1 | Varicellovirus Genus |
| Glanders | Farcy | Burkholderia mallei |
| Equine Viral Arteritis | EVA | Arterivirus Genus |
| Japanese Encephalitis | JE | Flavivirus Genus |
| Trypanosoma | Surra | T. evansi |
| Venezuelan equine encephalomyelitis | VEE | Alphavirus Genus |
| Tularemia | Rabbit Fever | F. tularensis |
| West Nile Fever | WNF/WNV | Flavivirus Genus |

Porcine

| | | |
|---|---|---|
| Foot and Mouth Disease | FMD | Orbivirus (22 species) |
| Vesicular Stomatitis | VS | Visiculovirus Genus |
| Swine Vesicular Disease | SVD | Enterovirus |
| Rinderpest | RP | Morbillivirus Genus |
| African Swine Fever | ASF | Asfivirus |
| Classical Swine Fever | Hog Cholera | Pestivirus |
| Nipah virus encephalitis | NVE | Henipahvirus Genus |
| Anthrax | Wool Sorters Disease | B. anthracis |
| Aujesky's Disease | Pseudorabies | Varricelovirus Genus |
| Echinococcus | Hydatidosis | E. granulosus |
| Leptospirosis | Weil's Disease | L. interrogans |
| Rabies | Mad Dog Disease | Lyssaviruses Genus |
| Trichinella | Trich | T. spiralis |
| New World Screwworm | Screw-worm | C. hominivorax |
| Old World Screwworm | Screw-worm | C. bezziana |
| Cysticercosis Pork | Tapeworm Disease | T. solium |
| Swine Brucellosis | Bang's Disease | B. suis |
| Transmissable gastroenteritis | TGE | Coronovirus Genus |
| Porcine reproductive & respiratory syndrome | PRRS | Arterivirus Genus |
| Japanese Encephalitis | JE | Flavivirus |
| Tularemia | Rabbit Fever | F. tularensis |

Poultry

| | | |
|---|---|---|
| Highly pathogenic avian influenza | AIV | Influenza Virus A |
| Low pathogenic avian influenza H5 or H7 | AIV H5 | Influenza Virus A |
| Newcastle Disease (Exotic) | ND | Avulavirus Genus |
| Turkey Rhinotracheitis | Avian Metapneumovirus | Pneumovirus Genus |
| Avian Infectious Bronchitis | AIB | Coronovirus Genus |
| Avian Infectious Laryngotracheitis | AIL | Varicellovirus Genus |
| Duck Viral Hepatitis | DVH | Avihepatovirus Genus |
| Fowl cholera Avian | Cholera | P. multocida |
| Fowl Typhoid | Typhoid | S. gallinarum |
| Infectious Bursal Disease | Gumboro Disease | Avibirnavirus genus |
| Marek's Disease | Marek's | Gallid herpesvirus 2 |
| Mycoplasmosis Avian | Infectious Anemia | M. gallisepticum |
| Avian chlamydiosis | AC | C. psittaci |

| | | |
|---|---|---|
| Pullorum Disease | PD | S. pullorum |
| Mycoplasmosis Avian | Infectious Anemia | M. synoviae |

Aquaculture:
Fish

| | | |
|---|---|---|
| Viral Hemmorhagic Septicemia | VHS | Novirhabdovirus genus' |
| Spring Viremia of Carp | | Rhabdovirus carpio |
| Infectious Hematopoietic Necrosis | IHN | Novirhabdovirus Genus |
| Epizootic Hematopoietic Necrosis | EHN | Ranavirus Genus |
| Infectious Salmon Anemia | ISA | Isavirus Genus |
| Epizootic Ulcerative Syndrome | EUS | Aphanomyces Genus |
| Gyrodactylosis | | G. salaris |
| Red Sea Bream Iridoviral Disease | RSIVD | Seriola Genus |
| Koi Herpesvirus Disease | KHV | Herpesvirus Genus |

Mollusks

| | | |
|---|---|---|
| Infection | | B. ostreae |
| Infection | | B. exitiosa |
| Infection | | M. refringens |
| Infection | | P. marinus |
| Infection | | P. olseni |
| Infection | | X. californiensis |
| Infection with Abalone Herpes-like virus | AbHV | Haliotis Genus |

Crustaceans

| | | |
|---|---|---|
| Taura Syndrone | TS | Aparavirus Genus |
| White Spot Disease | WSSD | Penaeus japonicus (contrib) |
| Yellowhead Disease | YD | Okavirus Genus |
| Infectious hypodermal/haematopoietic necrosis | IHR | Brevidensovirus Genus |
| Crayfish Plague | CP | A. astaci |
| Infectious myonecrosis | IM | Giardiavirus Genus |
| White Tail Disease | WTD | Whispovirus Genus |
| Necrotizing Helatopancreatitis | NHP | Vibrio Genus |

# INDEX